about the author

Judy Ghapman is the author of the bestselling *Aromatherapy Recipes for Your Oil Burner,* published by HarperCollins in 1998.

Always drawn to the world of beauty, design and natural healing, she created and co-founded the aromatherapy-based 'Sanctum Pure Body Product' range in 1990. From here Judy moved on to work as PR/Communication Manager for Australia's largest environmental education organisation, Planet Ark.

Judy lives in Byron Bay, Australia, and is a columnist for *Pure* magazine. This is her second book.

photography by Robert Reichenfeld

styling by Jane Collins

MORE Aromatherapy

recipes from around the world

judy chapman

Thorsons

Thorsons
An imprint of HarperCollin*Publishers,* Australia

First published in Australia in 2001
Reprinted in 2001
by HarperCollins*Publishers* Pty Limited
A member of the HarperCollins*Publishers* (Australia) Pty Limited Group
www.harpercollins.com.au

HarperCollins*Publishers*
25 Ryde Road, Pymble, Sydney, NSW 2073, Australia
31 View Road, Glenfield, Auckland 10, New Zealand
77-85 Fulham Palace Road, London W6 8JB, United Kingdom
Hazelton Lanes, 55 Avenue Road, Suite 2900, Toronto, Ontario M5R 3L2
and 1995 Markham Road, Scarborough, Ontario M1B 5M8, Canada
10 East 53rd Street, New York NY 10022, USA

National Library of Australia Cataloguing-in-Publication data:

Chapman, Judy, 1967– .
    More aromatherapy recipes from around the world.
    Includes index.
    ISBN 0 7322 7135 5.
    1. Aromatherapy. I. Title
668.542

Cover and internal photography by Robert Reichenfeld. Styling by Jane Collins
Cover and internal design by Judi Rowe, HarperCollins Design Studio
Printed in Hong Kong by South China Printing Co. on 115gsm Impress Art
7 6 5 4 3 2   01 02 03 04

contents

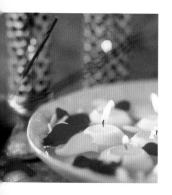

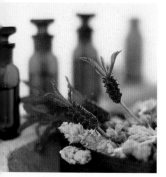

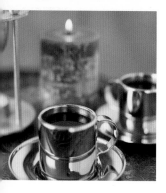

about aromatherapy

The future of this world looks so beautiful. As we dig our toes deeper into the earth and take conscious steps to care for our planet, our friends and ourselves, our inner light will shine. We are all connected to each other and to nature. As we realise this and come to respect our own wellbeing, and give this knowledge to others, the snowball effect will be awesome. We will be overcome with joy. Embracing nature in all its forms is the key to finding our own love, and aromatherapy is just one superb way to bring us back to the source.

The recipes in this book are designed to bring the world together and celebrate all the variations of plants and flowers that echo the uniqueness existing in different cultures. Wherever possible, the recipes are created with oils cultivated from that area. Where that is not possible, the oils reflect the energy and beauty of that place. One of the greatest pleasures of aromatherapy is creating your own personal blends. Another source of inspiration is exploring the aromas you like and studying their healing properties.

One of the things that motivated me to write this book was the desire to show how nature grows wild across the planet and humankind's journey to heal and rejuvenate using plants and flowers. I wanted to bring the world together under the umbrella of aromatherapy—to show that the differences in cultures are here to be celebrated.

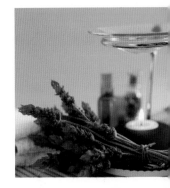

Plants are the source of medicine, and we continue to search for experiences and substances that will help alleviate pain and enhance joy and calmness. The art of aromatherapy involves the use of essential oils derived from specific plants, roots, barks, leaves, flowers and fruit. These are considered the 'life force' and heartbeat of the plant; the essences extracted are absolutely alive and vital. Essential oils are used like therapy to affect our mind and body through massage, compresses, bathing, cosmetics, perfumes and, as we explore in this book, through vaporisation.

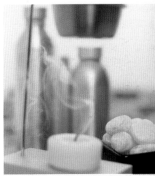

From ancient writings and Chinese manuscripts we have learnt that priests and physicians were using essential oils thousands of years ago. The Egyptians are believed to be the first people to discover the

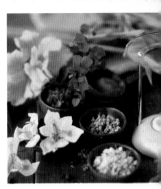

potential of fragrance and were luxuriating in the aromas of plants as far back as the golden age in the 12th Dynasty. They used plants and flowers in recipes for cosmetics (henna for hair, kohl for mascara), as well as in rituals, ceremonies and for medicine. These preparations included myrrh, frankincense, cedarwood and juniper, and were found well preserved in ivory boxes, jars, bottles and vases in Egyptian tombs. Around the same time, the Greeks were using herbs for medicine, as revealed in the recipes for medicinal perfumes inscribed on marble tablets in Greek temples. Hippocrates, the 'father of medicine', explored aromatics, including aniseed and fennel, medicinally. Meanwhile, in the east, the Chinese were exploring the use of plants along with acupuncture. However, it is the Arabians who seem to have discovered the art of distilling the essential oil from plants, with their first experiments done on the rose flower. Later, the Europeans began bathing in perfumes of clove, cinnamon, pine and frankincense.

Our experience of scent is due to the subtle layering effect of all the 'notes' of a compound as they blend into the atmosphere. The ability to smell is actually our most powerful sense. If you think about it, we are often attracted to people because of the way they smell, and certain smells trigger impressions, feelings and memories—our 'scent memory'. When we inhale a fragrance, the smell itself directly activates the limbic system, cortex and other areas of the brain that control impulses such as hunger and our emotions, and we have the ability to store over 10,000 different smells. The 'intelligence' of essential oils is incredible. They can be used to deliberately and effectively reach parts of the brain that influence our emotional state.

Essential oils are extracted using different methods, including steam distillation. In this method, the oil-giving part of the plant is placed inside a stainless steel distillation vat where the extreme steam pressure breaks down the plant material, releasing the essential oil from the plant cells. When cooled, the oils evaporate naturally from the water. The residual water is used for cosmetic purposes. Floral waters such as Orange Blossom and Rosewater make wonderfully hydrating and refreshing splashes for the face and body and can also be used in the oil burner.

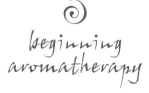

beginning aromatherapy

The way we select our essential oils is vital. Like in the food industry, there are oils that are produced organically and with great care, and others that are mass-produced from plants on which fertilisers and pesticides have been used. Naturally, the way an essential oil is produced does have an effect on its quality and healing potential.

When selecting essential oils, choose those labelled '100% pure essential oil' which have been packaged in dark glass and, preferably, stored in a cool, dark area. Some oils, such as Jasmine and Rose, are usually only available

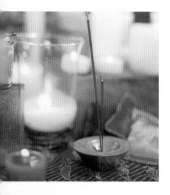

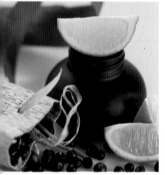

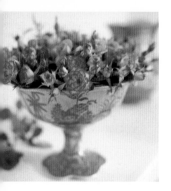

diluted at five per cent in a carrier oil due to the cost of the oil. As long as it is clear that the Jasmine is still a pure oil, its aromatherapeutic qualities will be effective.

Never buy essential oils that are packaged in clear glass or any plastic, and always store your oils away from heat and moisture (for example, not in the bathroom). The ideal aromatherapy accessory for oils is a wooden storage box.

The recipes in this book are only for blends to use in your oil burner. An aromatherapy kit consists of an oil burner or vaporiser, small tea-light candles and essential oils of your choice. An oil burner is normally a two-tiered structure with a dish at the top to hold the water and essential oil blend, and a surface below on which the candle rests. It is best to use an oil burner with a ceramic dish to prevent the oils from impregnating the dish permanently with an aroma. Fill the dish with water and light the candle. When the water has been warmed, add the drops of essence and allow the aromatherapy experience to unfold.

Enhance your day with the simple magic of aromatherapy. When a friend has a headache, massage their temples with a base oil containing a few drops of pure Peppermint oil. Or run a bath for them and add some Lavender droplets. Or vaporise a blend containing Lavender in an oil burner. There is really no limit to how many drops of oil you can blend, but six to eight is generally plenty.

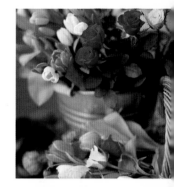

Through aromatherapy, we can stay connected to the source. Like the serene presence of the tall sandalwood tree itself, its aromatherapy oil can create calm and tranquillity. We can be instantly uplifted by the aromas of lime and lemongrass, evoking memories of travels through Thailand. The aromas of Africa can transport us back to wild journeys, the fragrances of Cuba can arouse sensual feelings and the smells of the Greek Islands can allow us to surrender to lazier moments.

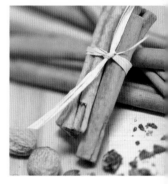

As we revive our trust in nature and embrace its wonders, our lives will be endless bubbles of joy.

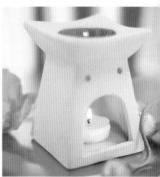

a note from the publisher

These recipes are to be used **purely for vaporising** (vaporising occurs when a few drops of an essential oil are added to warm water, heated in an oil burner, or vaporiser). Some essential oils can be harmful. Please take note of the following points:

- Never apply essential oils directly on your skin.
- Never take essential oils internally.
- Discontinue the use of essential oils immediately if you suffer an allergic reaction, and seek professional advice.
- Never dilute more than a total of eight drops of essential oils in water for vaporisation, unless advised otherwise by a qualified aromatherapist.
- Always buy aromatherapy oils that are marked 100 per cent pure.
- Keep oils out of reach of children.

A number of aromatherapy oils can be **harmful to pregnant women**. If you are pregnant (or there is a chance you are pregnant) please refer to the glossary and consult a qualified aromatherapist, or your family doctor, before using any of the recipes in this book.

acknowledgements

This book was inspired mainly by my love for and addiction to travelling. That feeling of finding home in the places and spaces in between; the unknown, where my essence is nourished by the experience of immersing myself in other cultures and learning how others think, feel and live their lives.

I thank Katyi Denham with all my heart and gratitude for her help in creating beautiful recipes that transport you immediately to places visited or dreamed about. Your friendship and support during the last few years has been amazing.

Thanks to Alicia Amore for being available so spontaneously to model in the book. You are a part of my tribe! And Juliet Lamont for her editing contribution — I appreciate it so much.

As much as I would have loved to have visited all the places described in this book, I had to take the second-best route — via e-mail. Thank you to all my fellow gypsy friends from around the world for their help. The following people inspired me with their favourite places to live and visit. Davina Stephens, Adrienne Ferreria, Natalie Penn, Angela and Sally Matherick, John Killis, Darshan, Mia Rosen, Ralph Shultz and Ananda Cairns. I hope our paths keep meeting.

To the HarperCollins crew — especially Helen Littleton, Judi Rowe, Veronica Miller, James Herd, Cristina Rodrigues and Helen Johnson— and to Lucy Tumanow-West, photographer Rob Reichenfeld and stylist Jane Collins.

Finally, I give a big hug to those who supported me during the process of this second book. To my mother, CC, for morning cups of coffee and love — the race to the computer is over (or is it?), my beautiful sister Jessie for your grace, love and laughter, Dad, Liz, Sadhvi, Dyan, Adam Spinner, Louise Barry, Craig Saunders, Maya Sweeney, Kate Watt, Sam Lowe, Ku, Natalie Jaroc, Leah Wright, Zoe Walsh and Lucy Vader. You all keep my spirit grounded, my heart open and the miracle of my life flowering. Thank you!

Australasia

Ancient yet youthful.
Vast. Intuitive.
Relaxed.

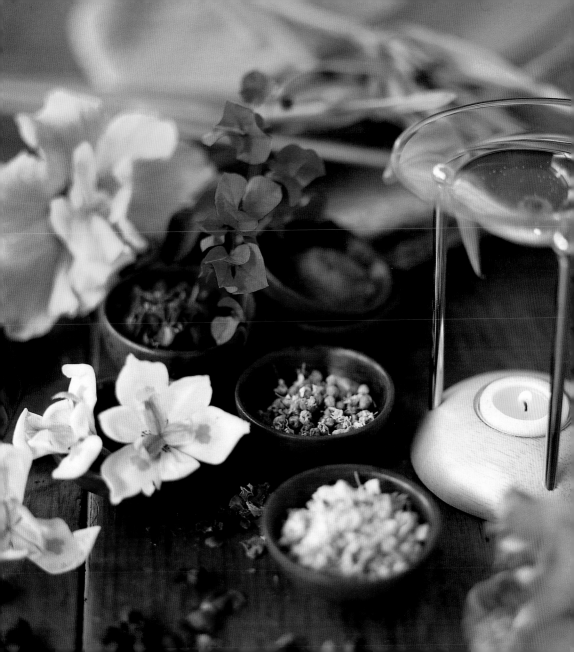

Inhale the aromas of these spacious and ancient lands. Living life to the fullest can be experienced here, where there is a mix of so many cultures living together and there is an abundance of breathtaking nature. Australia and New Zealand have a golden opportunity to lead the world into an age of total environmentalism. Relax and open up to all the beauty that surrounds you.

Australia

harmony

These blends create a calmer atmosphere and foster feelings of togetherness with oils known for their strong centring qualities. Moments of true harmony, such as when thousands of fellow Australians marched to say 'Sorry' to the indigenous people of Australia, serve to remind us that we are all family.

2 drops Cardamom
2 drops Lemon Myrtle
2 drops Tasmanian Lavender
or
2 drops Aniseed Myrtle
2 drops Lemon-scented Tea-tree
2 drops Western Australian Sandalwood

daintree

The lush rainforest growing in North Queensland is among the oldest in the world. The trees are strong and solid. The waters crystal clear. The rainforests provide an intense experience of nature for every traveller, and these grounding essences are to bring tranquility home to you.

2 drops Tea-tree

2 drops Cypress

2 drops Coriander

or

2 drops Cypress

2 drops Frankincense

2 drops Grapefruit

up north

Evoke the fragrance of a sultry summer, salt water, sand and fresh fruit with these essences. Recognised for their sensual qualities, they will bring a sense of excitement and delight to your day. Deliciously refreshing.

2 drops Ylang Ylang

2 drops Tea-tree

2 drops Cedarwood

or

2 drops Melissa

2 drops Patchouli

2 drops Juniper

mardi gras

The annual Mardi Gras celebration welcomes people from all over the world to one of Australia's biggest parties, where they are free to express themselves through dance and performance. To create your own vibrant atmosphere, burn these concoctions at gatherings and parties.

2 drops Grapefruit

2 drops Patchouli

2 drops Vetiver

or

2 drops Geranium

2 drops Sandalwood

2 drops Melissa

dreamtime

Blended to enhance inner wisdom and calm, these combinations of oils were inspired by the Aboriginal Dreamtime, where stories about nature, ancestors and animals are passed down through generations. The essence of Dreamtime is a connection with our earth.

2 drops Cajeput

2 drops Lemon

2 drops Bergamot

or

2 drops Fennel

2 drops Lavender

2 drops Sandalwood

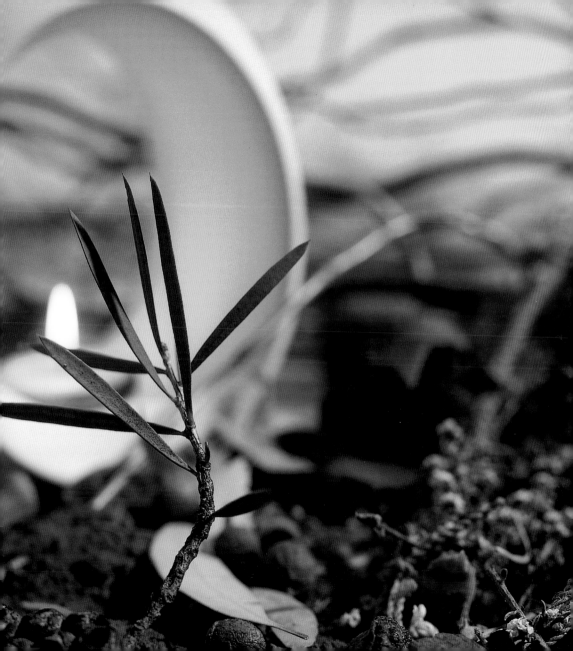

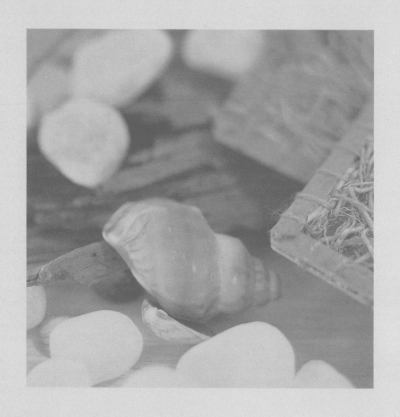

rushing river

Rivers mirror life: they flow, expand, narrow, change and surrender to the vast open seas. Clear and oxygen-rich Australian rivers rush over slippery rocks in the bush, refreshing everything in their path, just like these blends.

2 drops Lavender

2 drops Rosemary

2 drops Lemon-scented Tea-tree

or

2 drops Lemon Myrtle

2 drops Aniseed

2 drops Black Pepper

rainforest

Recreate the aliveness of an Australian rainforest and add an extra buzz to the room. The native Lemon Myrtle releases hits of lush citrus aromas when the foliage is crushed.

2 drops Lemon Myrtle

2 drops Sweet Marjoram

2 drops Patchouli

or

2 drops Lemon Myrtle

2 drops Nutmeg

2 drops Clary Sage

native breeze

Australia is home to hundreds of native plants and herbs that have been used in medicine and healing for centuries. Among them are the eucalypts, with their oil that is renowned for its antiseptic properties. The tangy, minty scent gives the air an uplifting yet cooling quality.

2 drops Peppermint Eucalyptus

2 drops Cedarwood

2 drops Bergamot

or

2 drops Citronella

2 drops Eucalyptus

2 drops Spearmint

ocean beauty

Seeing two humpback whales breach the ocean is an awesome experience. Equally amazing is swimming with dolphins in the sea. These blends evoke the ambience of the magical Australian oceans, ours to enjoy and take care of.

2 drops Lemon-scented Tea-tree

2 drops Peppermint

2 drops Rosemary

or

2 drops Melissa

2 drops Frankincense

2 drops Aniseed Myrtle

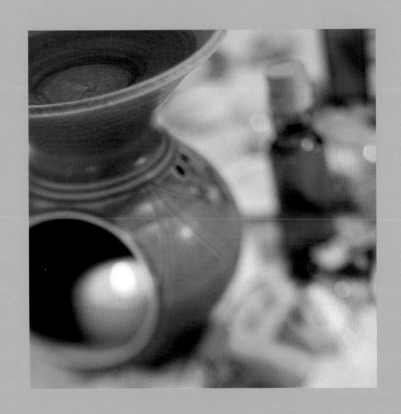

surf's up

When the surf's up, there's nowhere else to go. These blends of stimulating oils will enhance endurance, courage and vitality, so burn them when you're feeling fatigued and need some extra pep.

2 drops Orange

2 drops Patchouli

2 drops Clary Sage

or

2 drops Ginger

2 drops Frankincense

2 drops Chamomile

enchanted reef

These cleansing and energising blends reflect the vivid enchantment of the Great Barrier Reef. Their citrus explosions will lace the air with vigour, so make this a day for cleaning up your act and getting your life in order.

2 drops Lemongrass

2 drops Melissa

2 drops Chamomile

or

2 drops Bergamot

2 drops Basil

2 drops Lemon

heavenly sanctuary

The ultimate place to be—where you feel content, warm and secure. Create a heavenly sanctuary in your own home with soothing baths, healthy meals, heart-opening music and blends to burn for comfort and ease.

2 drops Ylang Ylang

2 drops Black Pepper

2 drops Vetiver

in Vanilla Water

or

2 drops Citronella

2 drops Bergamot

2 drops Lavender

spirit of uluru

Outback Australia has been host to many journeys of profound self-discovery. Inspired by the special spiritual significance of Uluru rising out of the surrounding vastness, these blends are ideal for creating a sense of expansion during times of personal growth.

2 drops Sweet Thyme

2 drops Marjoram

2 drops Lavender

or

2 drops Vetiver

2 drops Clary Sage

2 drops Ylang Ylang

rainbow magic

A place of celebration for indigenous Australians, magical Byron Bay attracts people from around the world who come to share the open and easygoing atmosphere. Conveying the same sense of paradise, these blends are to improve self-assurance, spirituality and vitality.

2 drops Aniseed Myrtle

2 drops Black Pepper

2 drops Geranium

or

2 drops Patchouli

2 drops Lemon Myrtle

2 drops Lime

natural healer

Indigenous Australians applied fresh leaves from the Tea-tree plant to wounds, and we still use the essential oils from these leaves for their medicinal properties. There are over 100 species blessed with these qualities. These blends bring freshness and clarity to a room, and stimulate healing.

2 drops Tea-tree

2 drops Cedarwood

2 drops Melissa

or

2 drops Tea-tree

2 drops Sandalwood

2 drops Clary Sage

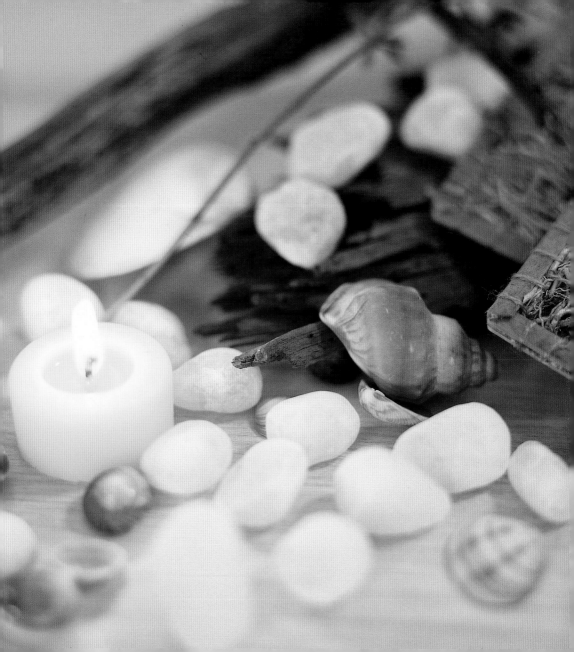

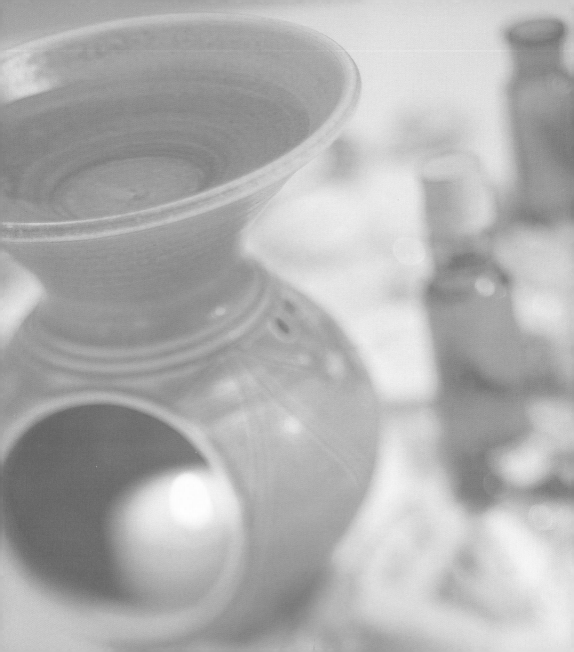

expansion

Fraser Island, off the coast of Queensland, is the largest sand island in the world, and spread across its centre are the deep, pure waters of Lake Mackenzie. Need to expand your horizons? Burn these blends and focus on your inner strength.

2 drops Nutmeg

2 drops Petitgrain

2 drops Clove

or

2 drops Juniper

2 drops Basil

2 drops Mandarin

southern calm

Known for its powerful relaxing and balancing properties, Lavender essence is distilled from the flowering tops of the plant. Whenever you're feeling anxious or burnt out, the delicate, sweet essence of Tasmanian Lavender will help you wind down and re-balance your emotional state.

2 drops Tasmanian Lavender

2 drops Clary Sage

2 drops Neroli

or

2 drops Tasmanian Lavender

2 drops Ylang Ylang

2 drops Vetiver

western serenity

Used in meditation and rituals since ancient times, Sandalwood is calming, enhances restful sleep, and helps relieve feelings of insecurity and loneliness. Use the essential oil of Western Australian Sandalwood for a local vibration in these serenity-making blends.

2 drops Western Australian Sandalwood

2 drops Cypress

2 drops Geranium

or

2 drops Western Australian Sandalwood

2 drops Patchouli

2 drops Lemon Myrtle

womad festival

Bring the world to your doorstep. WOMAD is a celebration of unity and friendship through dance and music. These fresh, aromatic blends will balance and ground you as dance and music does.

2 drops Lemongrass

2 drops Vetiver

2 drops Grapefruit

or

2 drops Vetiver

2 drops Clary Sage

2 drops Bergamot

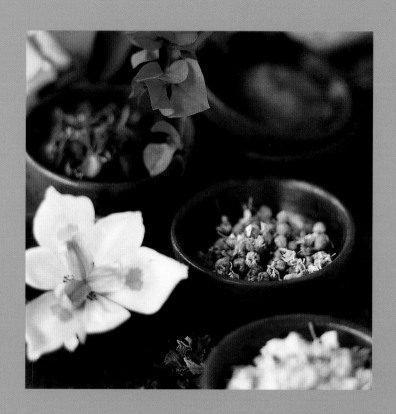

New Zealand

aotearoa

New Zealand, the 'land of the long white cloud', is surrounded by some of the most beautiful oceans in the world. Spending time near water is healing to the body and mind. Surround yourself with the serene and pure scents of the sacred, deep and unpredictable sea. Burn these blends to let your thoughts float away, and respect the sea and keep it clean.

2 drops Rosemary

2 drops Lavender

2 drops Cypress

or

2 drops Fennel

2 drops Lavender

2 drops Sandalwood

escape mode

New Zealand has so many mountains to climb, and so much ocean to dive in—so many retreats. When you're in need of a holiday or your appetite for life needs a boost, these stimulating blends will create a feeling of easy escapism.

2 drops Cypress

2 drops Coriander

2 drops Orange

or

2 drops Petitgrain

2 drops Vetiver

2 drops Sandalwood

chinatown

Celebrate the Eastern influences on Australian and New Zealand life with these exotic, spicy blends. Embrace the rich complexities of the aromas and the intermingling of cultures.

2 drops Nutmeg

2 drops Coriander

2 drops Frankincense

or

2 drops Cinnamon

2 drops Aniseed

2 drops Mandarin

café culture

Celebrate cosmopolitan life. Get that lively European café ambience in your living room next time you entertain. The energy of these essences will stimulate conversation and happy interaction.

2 drops Basil

2 drops Grapefruit

2 drops Rose Geranium

or

2 drops Lime

2 drops Ylang Ylang

2 drops Cedarwood

Asia

Balmy. Exotic.
Aromatic. Serene.

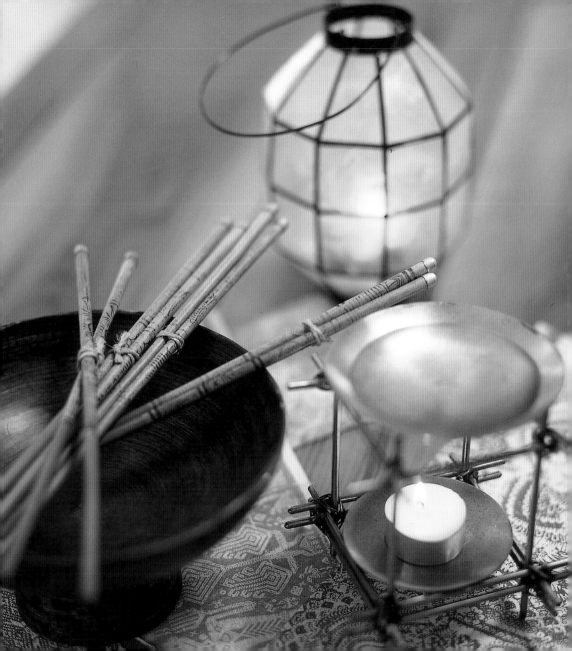

Eastern philosophies and practices of meditation and yoga can positively influence Western ways. They teach us the power of inner calm, no matter what surrounds us. Making the time to centre ourselves will give us an inherent grace. Let's immerse ourselves in the evocative aromas of the East.

Bali

sacred pura

The Balinese gracefully carry baskets of fruit and flowers on their heads, taking them as offerings to the *pura*, their temple. Experience moments of peace as you surround yourself with these delicate Eastern fragrances.

2 drops Ylang Ylang

2 drops Lemon

2 drops Nutmeg

or

2 drops Vetiver

2 drops Palma Rosa

2 drops Bergamot

the artist within

The town of Ubud is regarded as the artists' centre of Bali. The talented wood carvers and musicians live among the green rice paddies and work alongside the fantastic cafes. The entire scene is a sensory delight; a place where you can appreciate the simplicity of life. These blends are to inspire tranquility and looking within.

2 drops Ginger

2 drops Clove

2 drops Lemongrass

or

2 drops Orange

2 drops Bergamot

  in Vanilla Water

lotus café

The Lotus Café, in the town of Ubud, is famous for its beautiful pond filled with blossoming lotus flowers. Create the same impression of floral abundance with these blends and imagine yourself into a balmy Bali summer evening.

2 drops Ginger

2 drops Vetiver

2 drops Palma Rosa

or

2 drops Ylang Ylang

2 drops Black Pepper

2 drops Geranium

ceremony

The Balinese have a wonderful sense of ceremony. The incense, the gamelan music, the feasting, the joy. Create your own personal ceremony and allow goodness to filter into your life. Burn these blends, make some positive affirmations and turn your dreams into reality.

2 drops Sandalwood

2 drops Ylang Ylang

2 drops Palma Rosa

or

2 drops Nutmeg

2 drops Ginger

2 drops Lime

morning offering

The beautiful ritual of giving to the gods every morning is a Hindu tradition. The simple offerings include grains of rice, flowers and incense made from ground native roots and flowers. Bring a sense of joy and pleasure into your own life with these blends to burn in the morning.

2 drops Nutmeg

2 drops Ginger

2 drops Bergamot

or

2 drops Palma Rosa

2 drops Geranium

  in Rosewater

24

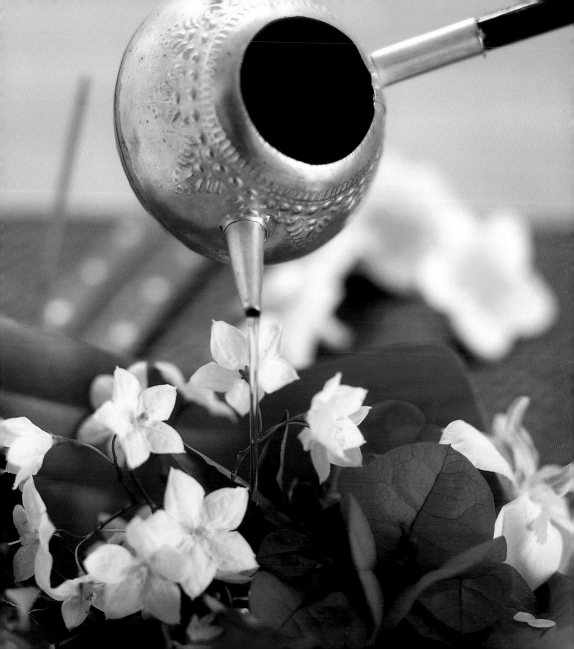

blue ocean

A favourite place for friends from all around the world to watch the sunset together, Blue Ocean beach has a truly magical atmosphere. A little lazy, a touch aphrodisiacal, these blends make for a similarly tantalising summer evening.

2 drops Lime
2 drops Ylang Ylang
2 drops Black Pepper
or
2 drops Ginger
2 drops Rose Geranium
  in Vanilla Water

bali spa

Bali has many health spas and healing retreats. Recreate one in your own home. Take a luxurious bath, light some candles, and allow these aromas to take you to a place of deep relaxation.

2 drops Patchouli
2 drops Black Pepper
2 drops Nutmeg
or
2 drops Nutmeg
2 drops Ginger
2 drops Ylang Ylang

Japan

blossom time

The traditional Japanese sense of fashion and design goes hand in hand with the people's grace and beauty. They also have incredible respect for their health, with a diet of seaweed, rice, fish and green tea. Create the delicate and fresh aromas of blossom time in the Japanese spring, and take time to ponder your own sense of self.

2 drops Cinnamon

2 drops Geranium

2 drops Neroli

or

1 drop Black Pepper

2 drops Ylang Ylang

1 drop Geranium

  in Vanilla Water

shinto chi

Appreciation of life and the people you are surrounded by is the essence of shinto, the original Japanese culture; seeing the world through optimistic eyes, believing that the spirit of life exists in the mountains, seas, rocks, rivers and trees. Celebrate the richness of your life and those close to you with these blends.

2 drops Cedarwood

2 drops Sandalwood

2 drops Orange

or

2 drops Lemon

2 drops Bergamot

2 drops Clary Sage

temple

There are thousands of temples in Japan, but the most valued is the body. To love and respect your own body is a positive step toward a healthier and happier life. Begin by burning these cleansing and purifying essences to refresh and uplift the atmosphere.

2 drops Cedarwood

2 drops Sandalwood

2 drops Orange

or

2 drops Lemon

2 drops Bergamot

2 drops Clary Sage

zen

Get back to the basics of life and ground your emotions. These blends are good to burn when you're feeling off-centre and anxious. Zen is all about going with the flow; being clear, present and open.

2 drops Lime

2 drops Juniper

  in Orangeflower Water

or

2 drops Aniseed

2 drops Lime

2 drops Cedarwood

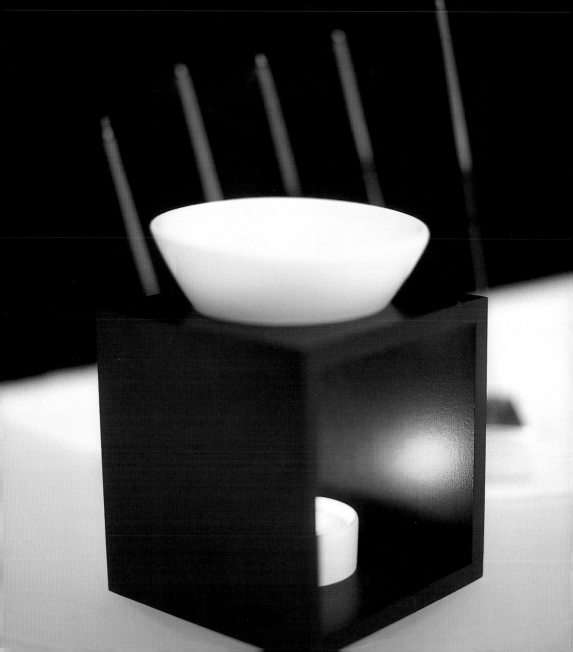

bodhi dharma

Celebrate non-violence, tolerance and compassion with these blends and bring a sense of peace into the room. Burn them when you need to be more honest with yourself and to express your truth to others. Take a deep breath and let your honesty flow.

2 drops Petitgrain
2 drops Clary Sage
  in Vanilla Water
or
2 drops Juniper
2 drops Aniseed
2 drops Geranium

tokyo steam

A fast-paced city, alive with ambition, Tokyo is an international centre for high achievement. Come alive with these stimulating oils selected to increase motivation and sense of direction, especially when you're facing a challenging task.

2 drops Bergamot

2 drops Black Pepper

2 drops Clary Sage

or

2 drops Geranium

2 drops Aniseed

1 drop Peppermint

samurai

There are times in our lives when we need to express our warrior side; to take a deep breath and be brave in what we do, to face situations we might have been avoiding, and not let others put us down. These blends are ideal when you need extra courage and vitality.

2 drops Juniper

2 drops Cinnamon

2 drops Lime

or

2 drops Peppermint

2 drops Orange

2 drops Aniseed

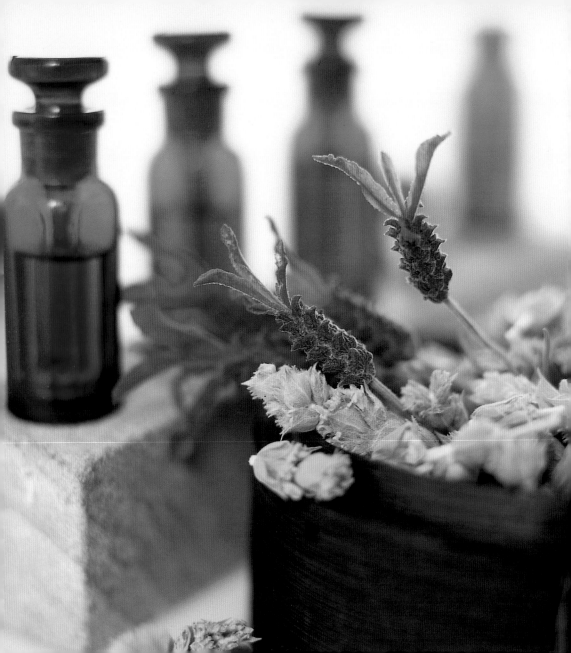

japanese bath

The *onsen*, or bath, is central to the Japanese notion of health and beauty. Burn these calming preparations while you soak in your bath after a challenging day's work.

2 drops Neroli

2 drops Lavender

2 drops Geranium

or

2 drops Bergamot

2 drops Patchouli

2 drops Palma Rosa

geisha girl

Let your love shine through in response to your lover's touch. Burn these blends to heighten sensuality and self-love, and bathe in the aromas of your personal pleasure dome. You deserve the utmost appreciation and attention from your partner.

2 drops Juniper

2 drops Neroli

2 drops Bergamot

or

2 drops Vetiver

2 drops Petitgrain

2 drops Ginger

India

ayurveda

Ayurveda, an ancient Hindu medical approach using herbs and massage, is an important part of health maintenance in the Indian culture. How you think and feel is reflected in your energy levels, and the way you carry and hold yourself. Burn these energising blends and invite joy and spontaneity into your life.

2 drops Geranium

1 drop Cardamom

2 drops Coriander

1 drop Lime

or

2 drops Orange

2 drops Geranium

2 drops Cardamom

buddha hall

In India, you can go to Buddha Hall and dance until your spirit soars. Guaranteed to thaw a cold heart and open up locked-in emotions, these blends will help to give you the strength to allow yourself to feel again.

2 drops Sandalwood

2 drops Cardamom

2 drops Lime

or

2 drops Ginger

2 drops Patchouli

2 drops Rose

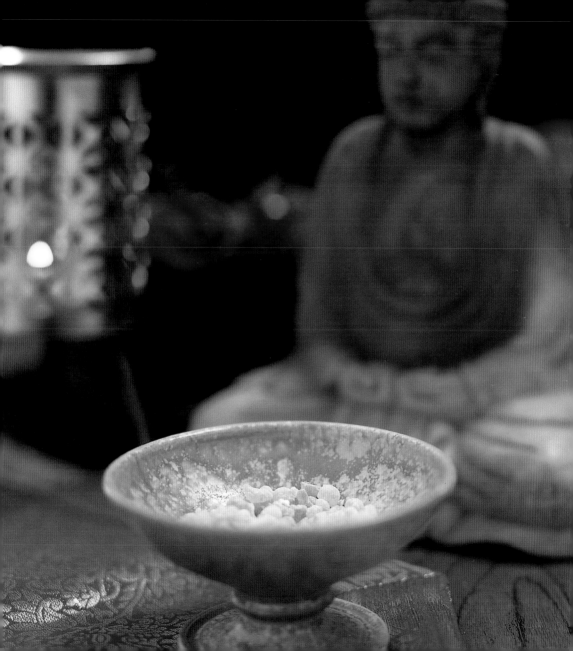

shanti shanti

Chill out, take it slowly, don't rush, and you may find your journey through life will be all the richer. The really exquisite moments in life are often those experienced in nature and shared with loved ones. Take time out from the quest for money and success to enjoy life in its simplicity. Burn these blends to aid your life journey.

2 drops Sandalwood

2 drops Myrrh

2 drops Clary Sage

or

2 drops Sandalwood

2 drops Cardamom

in Orangeflower Water

malabar wave

Crazy and chaotic, the city of Mumbai has a heady atmosphere that's hard to resist. As is the sophistication of the Malabar Hills. These hot and spicy blends are not for the faint-hearted.

2 drops Black Pepper

2 drops Jasmine

2 drops Patchouli

or

2 drops Jasmine

2 drops Bergamot

2 drops Neroli

in Vanilla Water

goa magic

Portuguese architecture and a unique quality of light contribute to the magic of Goa. People come from all over the world to experience a mind-shift, dancing all night on moonlit beaches and luxuriating in the gentle hospitality of the elegant Goanese. Burn these blends when you want mellowness and ease to reflect the pace of this place.

2 drops Indian Rose

2 drops Myrrh

2 drops Coriander

or

2 drops Jasmine

2 drops Sandalwood

2 drops Cardamom

candolim beach

A secluded Goan escape with cafes along sandy beaches, palm trees and starry skies. At sunset, drummers play, and at sunrise, people meditate. These are delicate aromas to create an easygoing ambience.

2 drops Jasmine

2 drops Geranium

2 drops Cardamom

  in Rosewater

or

2 drops Black Pepper

2 drops Vetiver

2 drops Geranium

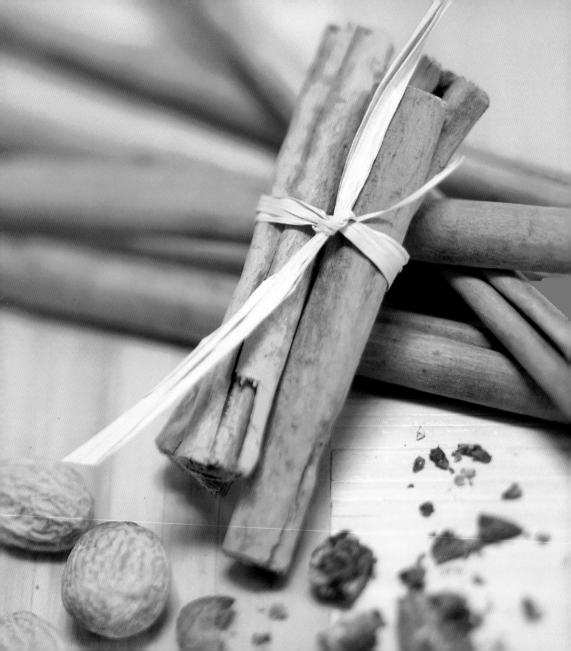

cinnamon stick

Warm, spicy and sweet is the flavour of cinnamon cultivated in India. It comes from the bark of the tree, and is one of the earliest spices to be used in cooking and medicine. Beautifully soothing when you're feeling overwhelmed and tired. Exotic and evocative.

2 drops Cinnamon

2 drops Ginger

2 drops Nutmeg

or

2 drops Cinnamon

2 drops Geranium

2 drops Vetiver

jaipur

The past comes alive in a place like Jaipur, rich with vivid colours and fascinating legends. These blends will weave a tapestry of intrigue with a dash of romance. Recline and dream of Jaipur.

2 drops Coriander

2 drops Sandalwood

2 drops Jasmine

or

2 drops Neroli

2 drops Indian Rose

2 drops Ginger

satori

Be seduced by the unknown.
Surrender to the path of no time,
and live moment to moment. The
challenge in life is to know that
wherever you are, you created it,
and that whatever you do, do it
with grace, honesty and care.
These aromas will relax and
calm you.

2 drops Jasmine

2 drops Marjoram

2 drops Coriander

or

2 drops Frankincense

2 drops Myrrh

2 drops Jasmine

samsara

Samsara is the endless cycle of
birth, death and rebirth in Hindu
belief, and these blends are ideal to
burn when you are starting a new
job or relationship, or going on a
journey. The oils are to enhance
positivity and provide inner comfort.

2 drops Geranium

2 drops Jasmine

2 drops Ginger

or

2 drops Black Pepper

2 drops Jasmine

2 drops Ginger

nirvana

The final release from the cycle of reincarnation, nirvana is attained by the extinction of all desires. Nirvana is stillness; it is being without the need to look any further than yourself for contentment. An aromatic splice of spice, these blends are calming when you're feeling discomfort or anxiety.

2 drops Clove
2 drops Jasmine
2 drops Neroli

or

2 drops Jasmine
2 drops Patchouli
2 drops Coriander

pearl of the orient

Cinnamon, black pepper and citronella are cultivated on the mango-shaped island of Sri Lanka, also known as the Pearl of the Orient, to be used to make essential oils. This delicious selection of revitalising oils will bring the fresh scent of nature to the room. Incredibly uplifting.

2 drops Cinnamon

2 drops Geranium

2 drops Lemongrass

or

2 drops Black Pepper

2 drops Lemongrass

2 drops Ginger

sandalwood serenity

Thousands of people go to the city of Mysore each year to study and practise yoga. The city itself is memorable for the smell of sandalwood incense filtering through the streets. Offering deep restfulness, these blends are perfect when you want to create a placid environment.

2 drops Mysore Sandalwood

2 drops Cardamom

2 drops Geranium

or

2 drops Sandalwood

2 drops Coriander

2 drops Patchouli

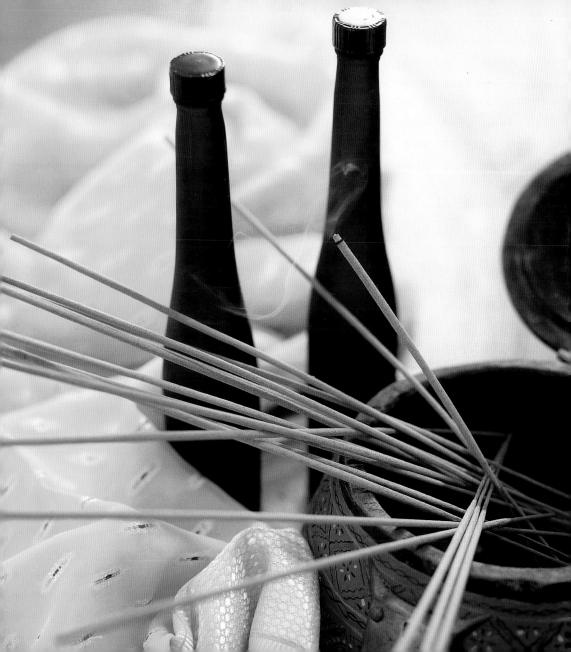

Tibet

tibetan chimes

Tibetans have a distinct culture with stunning expressions of creativity demonstrated in their sand mandalas and sculptures. These blends will keep the atmosphere uplifted and joyful. They are vibrant and positive mixes that will make for lightheartedness and playfulness.

2 drops Juniper

2 drops Sandalwood

2 drops Cinnamon

or

2 drops Cedarwood

2 drops Myrrh

2 drops Bergamot

himalayan skies

The Himalayas rise high above the world—a special place where time seems not to exist, but the significance of life is very much in focus. Burn these blends for moments of solitude and deep contemplation.

2 drops Jasmine

2 drops Juniper

2 drops Cedarwood

or

2 drops Coriander

2 drops Frankincense

2 drops Petitgrain

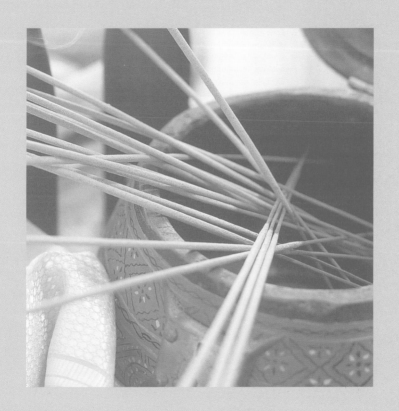

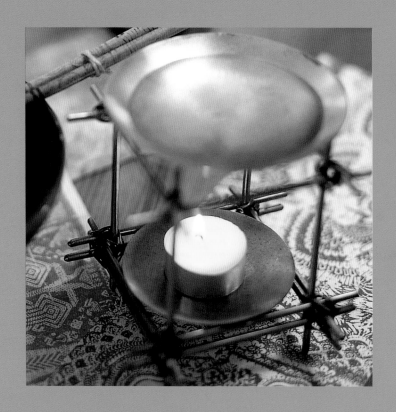

Vietnam

oc-om bo

This annual Vietnamese festival is held to give thanks for good crops and good health. At full moon, paper lanterns are released into the sky and banana-tree boats filled with offerings are floated downstream to music. Count your own blessings as you burn these uplifting yet relaxing blends.

2 drops Lemongrass

2 drops Geranium

2 drops Fennel

or

2 drops Geranium

2 drops Lemongrass

2 drops Mandarin

vietnamese vibrations

Tet is the Vietnamese tradition in which everyone makes a commitment to leave past problems and conflicts behind, and celebrate new beginnings with fireworks and dragons, and offerings of fruits, flowering peach trees and sweet rice cakes. These blends say: be brave and move on.

2 drops Cajuput

2 drops Geranium

2 drops Bergamot

or

2 drops Cajuput

2 drops Black Pepper

2 drops Lemon

Thailand

languid laos

North of Thailand, high in the mountains, is the special country Laos. These cooling blends will bring high altitude breezes on hot and humid days.

2 drops Basil

2 drops Lemongrass

2 drops Peppermint

or

2 drops Vetiver

2 drops Frankincense

2 drops Clove

thai fusion

Lush forests, jewel-like islands and bustling cities are all part of the Thailand experience, and all are beautiful in their own way. Lime and Lemongrass is a great combination if you are feeling fatigued or unfocused. Both of these invigorating blends are great for afternoon pep-ups.

2 drops Lime

2 drops Lemongrass

2 drops Ginger

or

2 drops Lemon

2 drops Neroli

2 drops Vetiver

moon fever

Celebrate in Thai style. At the Moon Fever festival, people let their hair down and dance until they can't any longer. Bring the beautiful aromas of Thailand into your room. These oils will create a sense of laughter and good times.

2 drops Grapefruit

2 drops Black Pepper

2 drops Ylang Ylang

or

2 drops Bergamot

2 drops Lime

2 drops Vetiver

my pen wry

A phrase you'll hear often in Thailand, *my pen wry* means 'don't worry'—relax, let it be. Thai people are known for their serene disposition. So, when the tension is rising, burn these blends and think *my pen wry*.

2 drops Coriander

2 drops Petitgrain

2 drops Sandalwood

or

2 drops Vetiver

2 drops Clary Sage

2 drops Rose Geranium

Indochine

indochine

The fading glory of French colonial architecture, the crumbling walls of ancient temples overtaken by glorious jungle growth—the triumph of nature. These green and serene blends will transport you to an Indochine state of mind.

2 drops Petitgrain

2 drops Bergamot

  in Rosewater

or

2 drops Petitgrain

2 drops Clary Sage

2 drops Geranium

les fleurs d'angkor

The 11th-century temple complex of Les Fleurs d'Angkor is surrounded by Cambodian jungle and has held people in awe for centuries. Indulge in wonder as you entertain great visions of your own, assisted by these enchanting blends.

2 drops Sandalwood

2 drops Petitgrain

2 drops Clary Sage

or

2 drops Ylang Ylang

2 drops Black Pepper

2 drops Frankincense

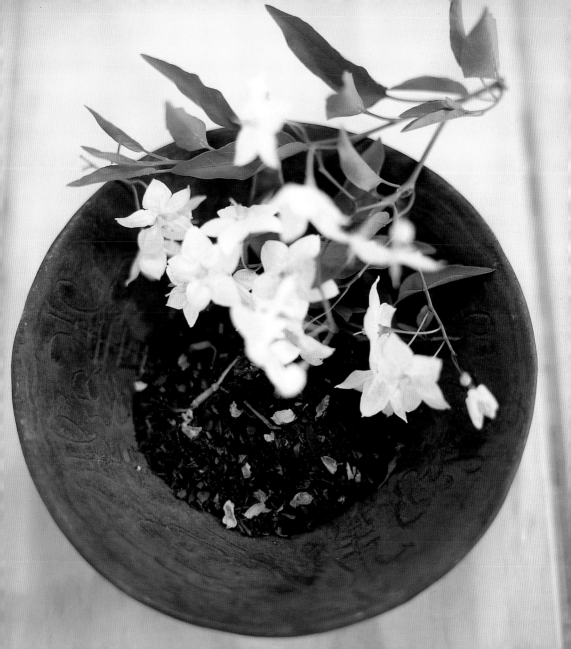

China

shanghai markets

Be motivated by the spicy fragrance of the Shanghai markets. These Eastern flavours are good to burn before a day of sport, movement or when you need extra energy.

1 drop Cinnamon

1 drop Black Pepper

1 drop Fennel

1 drop Clove

1 drop Star Anise

or

2 drops Star Anise

2 drops Cassia

2 drops Petitgrain

silk road

One of the first trade routes in China to link the East and West, the Silk Road was used by merchants who carried cargoes of silk, incense, spices and gems. Make your journey through life as smooth as silk. The Ginger in these blends has a warming and comforting effect. Take it easy.

2 drops Ginger

2 drops Geranium

2 drops Cardamom

or

2 drops Coriander

2 drops Ginger

2 drops Mandarin

jasmine infusion

The Jasmine flower releases a rich, sweet and musky aroma. It is used in China to scent tea and for hair decorations. It is also an expensive perfume ingredient—one of the most sensuous of all. Blended here with Asian essences, the infused Jasmine will create a special energy.

2 drops Geranium

2 drops Bergamot

2 drops Jasmine (infused)

or

2 drops Jasmine (infused)

2 drops Geranium

2 drops Juniper

ginger boost

The essence of Asia, Ginger is the best oil to burn when you're feeling a little stagnant and can't seem to break out of old patterns. Used in compresses to stimulate circulation, it may also help get your emotions moving. Its warming and spicy fragrance is especially wonderful on winter days.

2 drops Ginger

2 drops Star Anise

2 drops Geranium

or

2 drops Ginger

2 drops Cassia

2 drops Orange

Africa

Tribal. Rhythmic.
Imposing. Captivating.

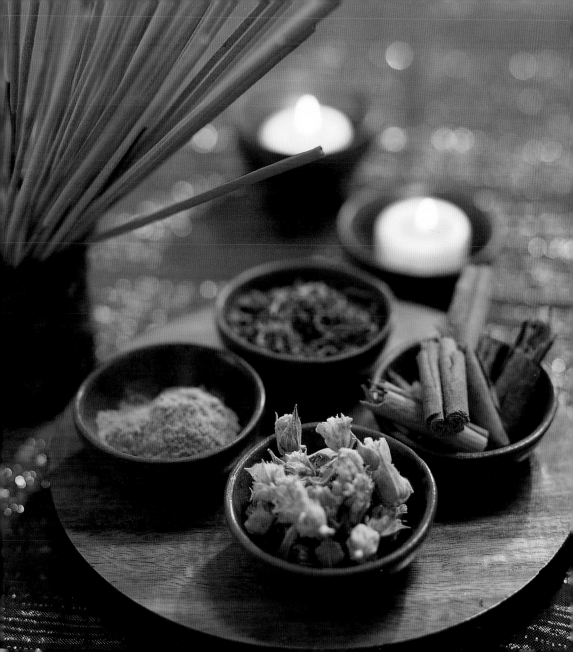

Be confident of who you are with the grounding essences of Africa. The beat of nature is celebrated here, where music and dance have influenced the rest of the world. Move out of your mind and into your body. Reach out to those around you with physical expressions of love to bring more warmth into your life.

afrodisia

Lying off the east coast of Africa is the magical island of Madagascar, where Ylang Ylang flowers bloom and their essence is distilled in the early morning. Where, too, music makes the world go around. Steeped in the soothing and aphrodisiacal effects of these blends, Madagascar won't seem so far away . . .

2 drops Ylang Ylang
2 drops Sandalwood
2 drops Neroli
or
2 drops Ylang Ylang
2 drops Frankincense
2 drops Geranium

african tang

Spiced for action, there is more than a hint of Africa in these confidence-boosting blends. Burn these potent combinations to motivate or empower yourself, and you'll be ready to take on anything.

2 drops Clove

2 drops Clary Sage

2 drops Nutmeg

or

2 drops Black Pepper

2 drops Frankincense

2 drops Palma Rosa

mosi-oa-tunya

Get into holiday mode instantly with these wonderful aromas. And remember, half the fun is in the planning, so start planning your next getaway now, always with something new and unexplored in your sights.

2 drops Lemongrass

2 drops Ylang Ylang

2 drops Fennel

or

2 drops Orange

2 drops Nutmeg

2 drops Chamomile

shaman

Africa is a land of contrasts: there are shimmering deserts, volcanoes and lush forests, as well as an abundance of wildlife. In touch with the rhythm of this land is the shaman, whose powerful healing abilities are at one with his natural environment. A true healer is often a friend who is not afraid to tell you the truth. These are soothing blends for difficult times.

2 drops Aniseed

2 drops Bergamot

2 drops Ylang Ylang

or

2 drops Neroli

2 drops Orange

2 drops Clove

moroccan midnight

A captivating North African country, Morocco is renowned for its evocative essences, including Cedarwood, Geranium, Myrtle, Star Anise, Chamomile, Petitgrain, Rosemary, Neroli, Rose and Jasmine Absolute. Create the aromas of this fascinating place with these recipes.

2 drops Myrtle

2 drops Geranium

2 drops Neroli

or

2 drops Cedarwood

2 drops Aniseed

2 drops Petitgrain

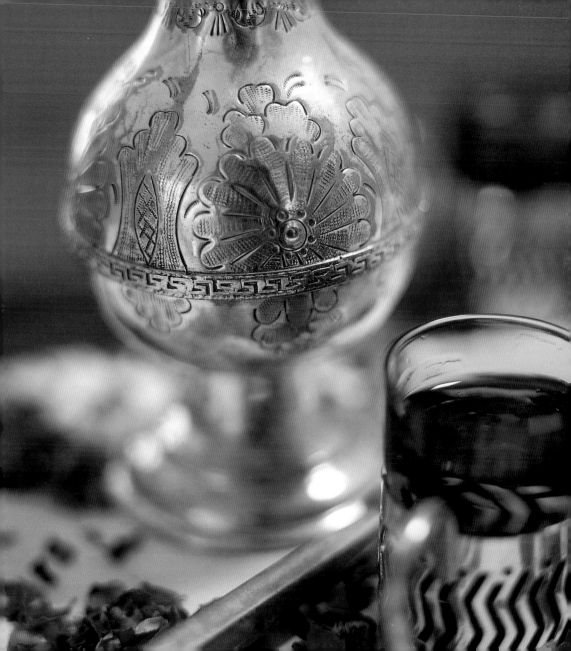

marrakesh

A magical city of palaces, romantic gardens, storytellers, herbal healers, Berber dancers, musicians and fire-eaters. Keep in mind that we are all on the journey and don't be too hard on friends going through unusual times. Mix up your own Marrakesh moment with these enchanting blends.

2 drops Frankincense

2 drops Cedarwood

2 drops Myrrh

or

2 drops Aniseed

2 drops Grapefruit

2 drops Patchouli

tangier

Perched on the tip of Africa, where the Atlantic Ocean melts into the Mediterranean, the Moroccan port of Tangier retains its aura of being a haven for the idealistic. These blends reflect the serenity of the setting.

2 drops Neroli

2 drops Myrtle

2 drops Chamomile

or

2 drops Cedarwood

2 drops Lemon

2 drops Chamomile

zanzibar zest

Off the east coast of Tanzania, this secret diamond of the Indian Ocean once produced most of the world's clove supplies. Other native spices grown there include cinnamon, nutmeg and pepper. The following blends create magnificent aromas with a warm and sensual feeling.

2 drops Clove

2 drops Clary Sage

2 drops Patchouli

or

2 drops Cinnamon

2 drops Clove

2 drops Orange

tribal spirit

African tribal rituals show an amazing synergy with, and respect for, the land and the animal and plant worlds. These aromatics will inspire a sense of friendship and harmony; an exotic blend of essences to stimulate the senses.

2 drops Black Pepper

2 drops Palma Rosa

2 drops Frankincense

or

2 drops Geranium

2 drops Rosemary

2 drops Lemon

sahara desert

The largest desert in the world, and covering over a quarter of Africa, the Sahara is a vast landscape of rocks, stones, evaporated ancient lakes, unpredictable winds and shifting sand dunes. A place of great beauty and power. Burn these blends when you need some Saharan solitude.

2 drops Frankincense

2 drops Fennel

2 drops Thyme

or

2 drops Sage

2 drops Cedarwood

2 drops Aniseed

casablanca

Another Moroccan city, this time with a cinematic reputation for love. The world definitely needs more heart. Come into each day with fresh, loving eyes. These blends were created with native essences to enhance the emotions of love and compassion. Perfect for creating a soft centre in which to sink with your loved one.

2 drops Bergamot

2 drops Chamomile

2 drops Geranium

or

2 drops Neroli

2 drops Nutmeg

2 drops Orange

arabian knights

The ancient city of Baghdad's stunning, intricate pink stone architecture echoes with tales of magic carpets and princesses. Affirm that your dreams are becoming a reality. Write down your goals for the coming year and reread them regularly. These are sensuous blends to evoke more excitement.

2 drops Cedarwood

2 drops Marjoram

2 drops Neroli

or

2 drops Cedarwood

2 drops Cardamom

2 drops Orange

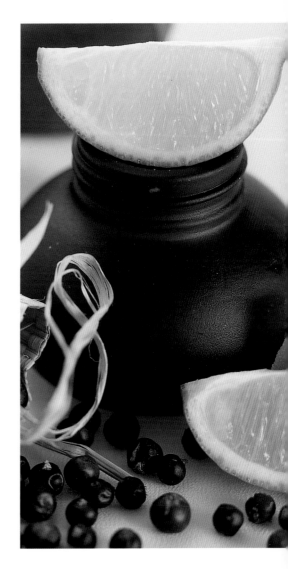

Egypt

egyptian incense

The Egyptians used these oils for their centring qualities. Take advantage of their effects when you are feeling indecisive and need a clear and quiet space. Make some time to breathe and think things through.

2 drops Geranium
2 drops Myrrh
2 drops Frankincense
or
2 drops Coriander
2 drops Marjoram
2 drops Sandalwood

cairo calling

This bustling city is surrounded by the calm and peaceful desert. Burn pure essences to conjure up the fragrances of Cairo, the musky scent that filters through the streets. Bring a sense of richness and liveliness to the air.

2 drops Coriander
2 drops Frankincense
2 drops Lemon
or
2 drops Peppermint
2 drops Clary Sage
2 drops Geranium

holy blends

The tale of the three wise men who came bearing gifts of gold, Frankincense and Myrrh reveals the value of these plants and flowers in ancient times. There are 188 references to aromatics in the Bible. Use this blend when you want to let go of the past and move forward with assurance.

2 drops Myrrh

2 drops Coriander

2 drops Geranium

or

2 drops Frankincense

2 drops Sandalwood

2 drops Black Pepper

isis

The Egyptian goddess Isis, divine mother and protector, was adored by the Romans who built many temples in her honour. Celebrate all the powerful gifts of the female gender, including highly developed intuition and natural openness. These delicate aromas are dedicated to the goddess.

2 drops Sandalwood

2 drops Clary Sage

2 drops Orange

or

2 drops Cedarwood

2 drops Geranium

2 drops Bergamot

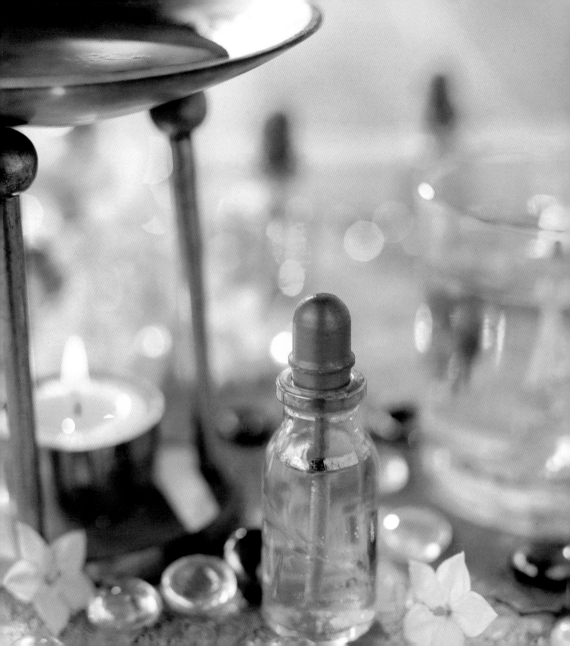

temple of luxor

This exquisite temple in the ancient
city of Thebes is a majestic sight.
Also exquisite is the presence of
love in a place. These blends are
beautiful to burn when you want
love flowing through a room. These
essences are to assist enhance
seduction.

2 drops Coriander

2 drops Ginger

2 drops Rose

  in Vanilla Water

or

2 drops Patchouli

2 drops Rose

2 drops Mandarin

garden of eden

Take a stroll through the Garden of
Eden with floral essences sourced
from nature. These aromas contain
balancing properties to calm and
centre.

2 drops Neroli

2 drops Lavender

2 drops Cedarwood

or

2 drops Neroli

2 drops Clary Sage

2 drops Coriander

queen of the nile

The Egyptian Queen Cleopatra lavishly used aromatic essences to lure her lovers. She even soaked the sails of her ship in Jasmine oil. When your lover visits, celebrate your shared souls with these alluring blends.

2 drops Jasmine

2 drops Bergamot

2 drops Sandalwood

or

2 drops Jasmine

2 drops Geranium

2 drops Neroli

cleopatra's perfumes

Fragrances are the result of centuries of research and refinement, passed down from generation to generation. Originally, all the finest perfumes were made by the Egyptians. Cleopatra's book on cosmetics and perfumery was particularly renowned. Plant essences were so valuable in those times, they were only used in temples and for royalty. These are four of Cleopatra's favourite fragrances, which have been recreated with some of the ingredients.

NOTE: These blends are NOT for topical application.

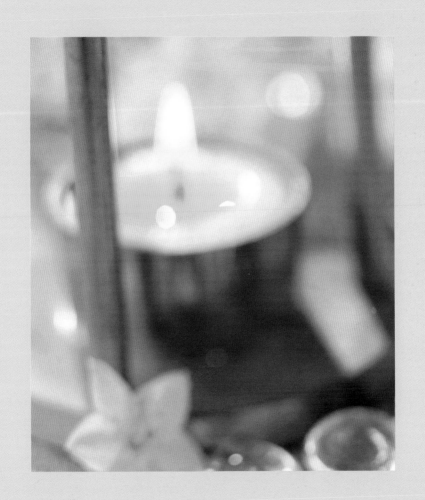

sunsinum—oil of the lilies

Made with ingredients including honey, Cinnamon, Myrrh and Saffron, Oil of the Lilies is an exquisitely delicate and feminine scent.

2 drops Cinnamon

2 drops Myrrh

2 drops Geranium

  in Vanilla Water

or

2 drops Cardamom

2 drops Ylang Ylang

2 drops Geranium

  in Vanilla Water

regale unquentum—royal oil

A powerfully exotic blend of essences, this perfume contained Myrrh, Rosewood, Marjoram plus spices and flowers brought from China, Malaysia and India.

2 drops Myrrh

2 drops Cedarwood

2 drops Ylang Ylang

  in Rosewater

or

2 drops Marjoram

2 drops Nutmeg

2 drops Geranium

  in Vanilla Water

rhodinum—oil of roses

Originally from Persia, this perfume was made with the essence of the beautiful rose flower.

2 drops Rose Otto

2 drops Palma Rosa

2 drops Geranium

or

2 drops Rose Damask

2 drops Bergamot

2 drops Rose Geranium

cyprinum—oil of cyperus reed

Created to appeal to men and women, this perfume included top notes of rejuvenating Lemongrass.

2 drops Cypress

2 drops Lemongrass

2 drops Clary Sage

or

2 drops Lemongrass

2 drops Cardamom

2 drops Geranium

Middle East

Moody. Intense.
Mysterious. Magical.

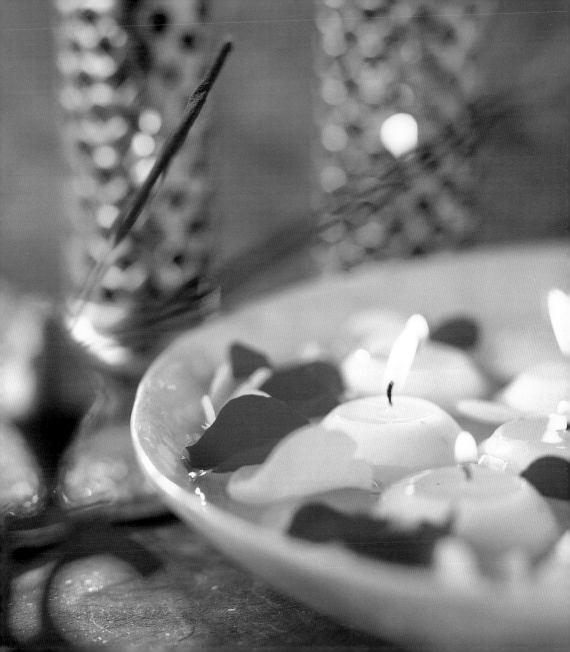

Surrender to the voices and visions from emerging generations that teach us that now is the time to let go of any past conflicts and move forward with global integrity. Life is so precious. The mixtures of cultures here can be experienced by the varying sounds of prayer echoing through the vast landscape. Be eager to love yourself and allow others to love you wholeheartedly.

deep spirit

Myrrh essential oil has deeply spiritual qualities and is used to enhance courage and willpower. It is distilled from the resin of the small, knotted Myrrh tree, whose white flowers can be seen blossoming in Arabian deserts. The smoky, balsamic aroma is soothing when fear and uncertainty prevail.

2 drops Rose

1 drop Myrrh

1 drop Vetiver

or

2 drops Sandalwood

2 drops Myrrh

2 drops Geranium

fountain of youth

People visit the Dead Sea for the healing and beautifying properties of the minerals its water and mud contain. Like a dip in the Dead Sea, these blends will bring out the best in you. Treat yourself with respect and love. Don't be afraid to show the world your utmost potential.

2 drops Neroli

2 drops Bergamot

2 drops Sandalwood

or

2 drops Clary Sage

2 drops Myrrh

2 drops Rose Geranium

arabian alchemy

The flower essences blended here capture the deep, musky aromas of Arabia that filter through the colourful bazaars. Avicenna was the Arab physician who, around the year AD 1000, researched over 800 plants and herbs for medicinal use, including the aromatics of Rose, Lavender and Chamomile. He also made major advances in the art of distilling.

2 drops Clove

2 drops Petitgrain

2 drops Geranium

or

2 drops Orange

2 drops Patchouli

2 drops Geranium

sufi elixir

These blends are to increase your inner strength and self-belief, especially in the face of decision-making. Take some time out to really think and feel things through. Trust yourself!

2 drops Myrrh

2 drops Frankincense

1 drop Sandalwood

or

2 drops Sweet Marjoram

2 drops Mandarin

2 drops Basil

ramadan

For 30 days in the ninth month of the Muslim year, strict fasting is observed from sunrise to sunset. At the end of the month, there is a feast. These blends capture the joy of cooking up a feast for loved ones—showing your gratitude for their love and support. A simple act such as this is a valuable gift.

2 drops Cedarwood

2 drops Coriander

2 drops Lime

or

2 drops Petitgrain

2 drops Ginger

2 drops Sandalwood

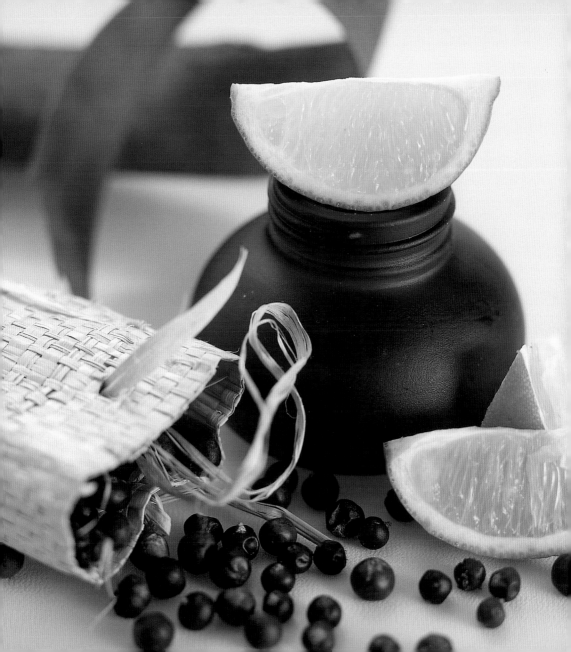

Israel

wild citrus

The evergreen lemon tree grows wild around Israel. The essential oil is expressed from the lemon peel. Burn these blends to give the room a sparkle, and when you are experiencing self-doubt or hazy thoughts, to bring joy and clarity to the air.

2 drops Fennel

2 drops Coriander

2 drops Lemon

or

1 drop Clary Sage

2 drops Lemon

1 drop Peppermint

city of gold

Jerusalem is known as the city of gold. It is a city of contrasts— ancient history and a cutting-edge future. Yin and Yang. Burn these strong and stimulating blends when you want to maximise the day's abundance. Spend a few moments visualising success in your mind.

2 drops Myrrh

2 drops Frankincense

2 drops Sandalwood

or

2 drops Geranium

2 drops Fennel

2 drops Sandalwood

sinai summer

A peninsula between the Gulfs of Suez and Aqaba, the special atmosphere of Sinai attracts an eclectic international crowd. Create the sense of endless relaxation with these blends when you just feel like being idle. To calm yourself, take a few breaths and think about all the good things that are happening in your life right now.

1 drop Black Pepper

2 drops Mandarin

2 drops Bergamot

or

2 drops Black Pepper

2 drops Ylang Ylang

1 drop Geranium

scents of solomon

The wise King Solomon of Israel is said to have written beautiful poetry with descriptions of aromatic herbs such as Myrrh, Lily, Rose, Cinnamon and Frankincense. These welcoming blends are to lift the mood of all who enter a room and inspire conversation, poetry and romance.

2 drops Mandarin

2 drops Cinnamon

1 drop Frankincense

1 drop Ginger

or

2 drops Rose

1 drop Myrrh

1 drop Coriander

2 drops Sandalwood

Mediterranean

Sparkling. Earthy.
Joyous. Confident.

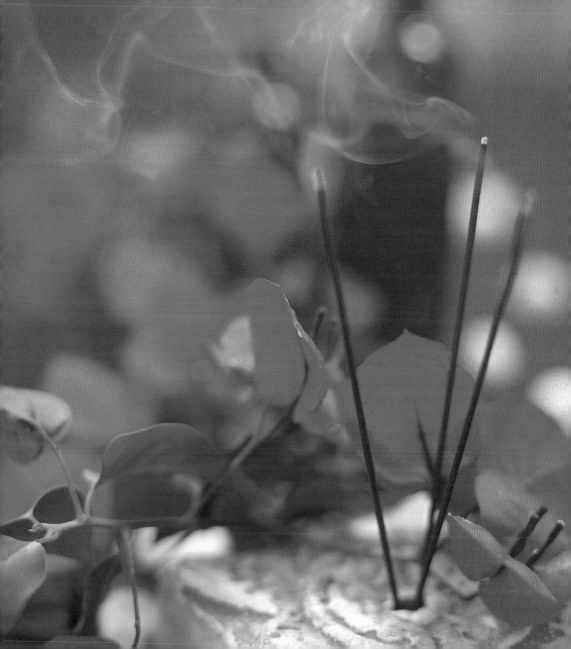

Enjoy the person you are and celebrate that you are alive. There is a very important reason why you exist – to have lots of fun and laughter. In the Mediterranean, people appreciate the finer things in life, such as food, wine and friends. Be seduced by aromas from Ibiza to Sardegna, and surrender to bliss.

Greece

siesta

The tradition of an afternoon siesta, where people rest for a few hours after a boisterous lunch with friends and family, is so civilised. Welcome the calming aromas of these blends known for their sedative properties. Solutions for anxious feelings, good for recovery.

2 drops Orange

2 drops Lavender

2 drops Bergamot

or

2 drops Chamomile

2 drops Sweet Marjoram

2 drops Fennel

sweet cheer

Marjoram grows wild throughout
the Mediterranean coastal region.
The essence is distilled from the
leaves and flowering tops of the
plant. It is highly regarded for its
positive effects on emotional grief
and loneliness, so burn it when
you're in need of warmth and hope.

2 drops Marjoram

2 drops Lavender

2 drops Bergamot

or

2 drops Marjoram

2 drops Rosemary

2 drops Cypress

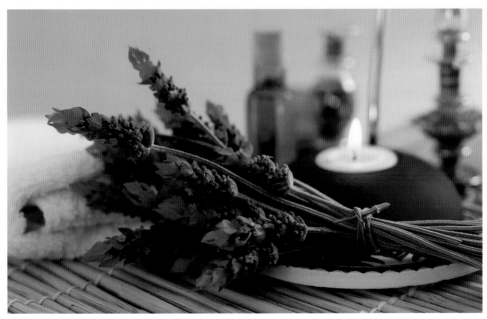

adonis

According to legend, handsome Adonis was said to have been born from the Myrrh tree. Loved by Aphrodite, he was worshipped for vegetation, fertility and rebirth. These blends will create a masculine aroma in the room, to celebrate the incredible beauty of men.

2 drops Lavender

2 drops Coriander

2 drops Cedarwood

or

2 drops Myrrh

2 drops Mandarin

2 drops Ginger

island odyssey

The Greek Islands culture is addictive: a simple, languorous lifestyle. Over 100 islands sparkle like sapphires in the sea. Make your life a jewel with plenty of days of peace and quiet. Burn these blends when you just want to sit around and talk, drink and devour delicious food.

2 drops Lemongrass

2 drops Sage

2 drops Thyme

or

2 drops Basil

2 drops Geranium

2 drops Bergamot

atlantis

The island of Santorini is believed to be the lost city of Atlantis, and when you stand on the cliffs, it is easy to see why. These breathtaking blends contain essences from nearby regions to bring vitality and a sense of delight to your day. Allow the mystery of life to unfold.

2 drops Melissa

2 drops Chamomile

2 drops Petitgrain

or

2 drops Geranium

2 drops Melissa

2 drops Lavender

mykonos recovery

Rediscovered by alternative travellers in the 1960s, the Greek island of Mykonos now attracts a wild international set who come to dance from sunset to sunrise. Burn these blends after too much indulgence and good fun. Recover in Mykonos style: chill out on the heavenly beaches.

2 drops Chamomile

2 drops Fennel

2 drops Lavender

or

2 drops Parsley

2 drops Hyssop

2 drops Lemon

sicilian specialty

The Italian island of Sicily has a character all of its own. Encourage the feeling of confidence and fulfilment with these blends created with Bergamot essential oil. Cold-pressed from peel of the rare citrus fruit, it releases a sweet and fruity scent, and is used for balancing the emotions. These are great blends for reducing anxiety and fear.

2 drops Bergamot

2 drops Cypress

2 drops Neroli

or

2 drops Bergamot

2 drops Clary Sage

2 drops Rose

aphrodite

The legend is that a poor Greek girl would visit the Greek temple of Aphrodite each morning with offerings of fresh flowers. One day, after a vision of the love goddess Aphrodite, she became a princess on the Persian throne. Don't undervalue what you know to be true in your heart, and use these blends to be in love with your life.

2 drops Cinnamon

2 drops Marjoram

2 drops Rose

or

2 drops Neroli

2 drops Rose

2 drops Cardamom

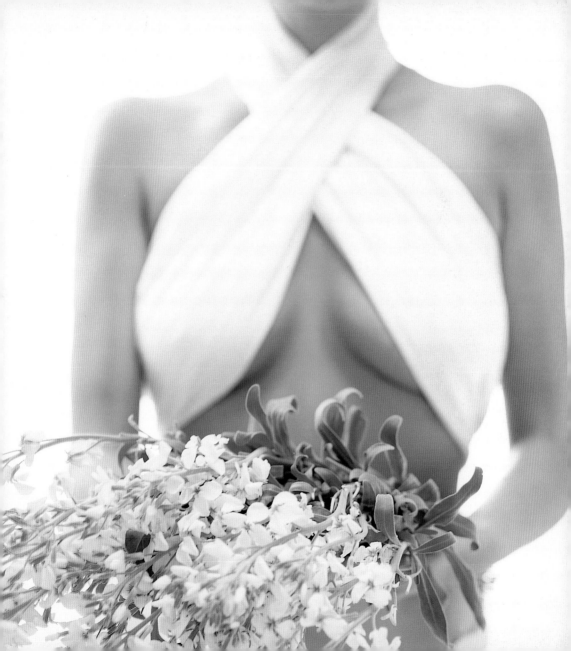

floral isle

The Greek island of Crete is known for its amazing ruins and attracts people interested in good health and rejuvenation. These blends carry the aroma of a delicate floral bouquet to reflect the island's 1,500 flower species. Create an energy of healing and esprit with these blends of aromatic oils.

2 drops Clary Sage

2 drops Petitgrain

2 drops Juniper

or

2 drops Hyssop

2 drops Clary Sage

2 drops Melissa

sardegna splash

Create a wild and sexy atmosphere to capture the essence of the beautiful Italian island of Sardegna. Enhanced by vast azure waters, this island is alive with energy. Burn these blends when you need zest in your day. Don't hold back; take a deep breath and let go.

2 drops Grapefruit

2 drops Pine

2 drops Rosemary

or

2 drops Cinnamon

2 drops Lavender

2 drops Peppermint

Portugal

viva rava

The climate and prevailing culture in Portugal tells you to kick off your shoes. The Cypress in these blends gives a pleasantly smoky, woody smell that reflects the seductiveness of the place. Burn these blends to strengthen your nerves during times of change.

2 drops Cypress

2 drops Fennel

2 drops Lemon

or

2 drops Cypress

2 drops Frankincense

2 drops Petitgrain

Ibiza

spanish quarter

The Spanish are loved for their lively and vivacious nature. Created with the essence of the Rosemary plant, which grows wild throughout Spain, these mixtures will enhance self-confidence and sexual energy. Let your emotions flow freely and you will feel naturally refreshed and healthier.

2 drops Rosemary

2 drops Orange

2 drops Cinnamon

or

2 drops Rosemary

2 drops Basil

2 drops Geranium

seville seduction

Courtyards of rose gardens and streets lined with orange trees paint this Spanish town with vivid colours while flamenco dancing adds dizzying motion. Made with essences to increase sensuality and passion, these blends will set off an explosion of romance in the air.

2 drops Orange

2 drops Rose

2 drops Melissa

or

2 drops Coriander

2 drops Melissa

2 drops Nutmeg

ibiza dreams

A Mediterranean island blessed with fig and orange trees, olives, almonds and pines, Ibiza is a haven for all kinds of people. Wind down with the help of these potions and create your own paradise with a dreamy and serene ambience. These are beautiful blends for summer evenings.

2 drops Pine

2 drops Geranium

2 drops Rosemary

or

2 drops Jasmine

2 drops Clary Sage

2 drops Pine

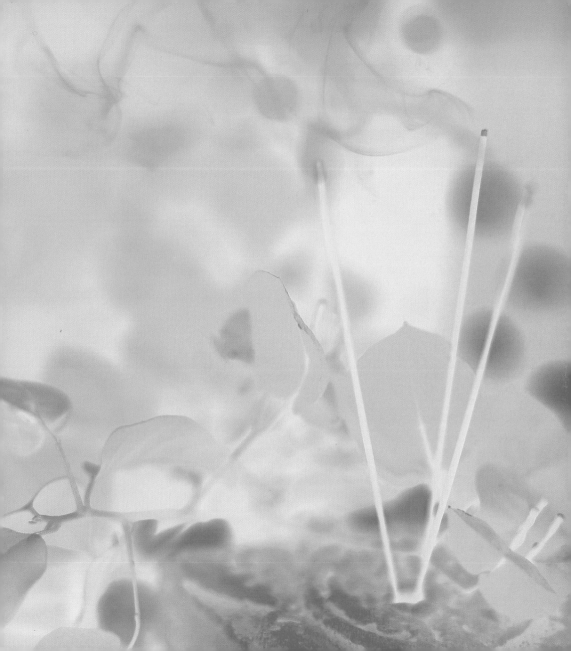

gypsy blood

The freedom to move on at will is a seductive aspect of the gypsy lifestyle. Don't lose sight of your own dreams and aspirations, and remember to take time out every now and then to re-evaluate your life purpose and your potential. For this moment, create a sense of mystery and unpredictability around yourself and lavish the atmosphere with these elusive yet irresistible aromas.

2 drops Cedarwood

2 drops Oregano

2 drops Orange

or

2 drops Geranium

2 drops Jasmine

2 drops Lavender

café del mar

The beauty of Ibiza lies in its alternatives—you can dance all night, or retreat to a secluded cove and experience intimacy with nature. Play some music and burn these blends to open your heart and enliven the air with a sense of idyllic romance.

2 drops Sage

2 drops Orange

2 drops Thyme

or

2 drops Clary Sage

2 drops Neroli

2 drops Vetiver

Southern France

cypress

An elegant and graceful tree that grows in the south of France, the Cypress releases a spicy and refreshing fragrance. Use it to rebalance and soothe when self-esteem is low. An ingredient in Tibetan incense, Cypress oil is useful when you need to accept changes happening in your life.

2 drops Cypress

2 drops Lemon

2 drops Bergamot

or

2 drops Cypress

2 drops Pine

2 drops Sandalwood

la croisette

Cannes' *La Croisette* is the star of the French Riviera, attracting exotic and creative people to the International Film Festival each year. These are decadent oils for special occasions, like today! Dedicate a portion of your day to self-indulgence: positive thoughts, delicious food or a soak in the bath.

2 drops Jasmine

2 drops Coriander

2 drops Sandalwood

or

2 drops Nutmeg

2 drops Neroli

2 drops Geranium

Europe

Exotic. Inspiring.
Grounded. Soulful.

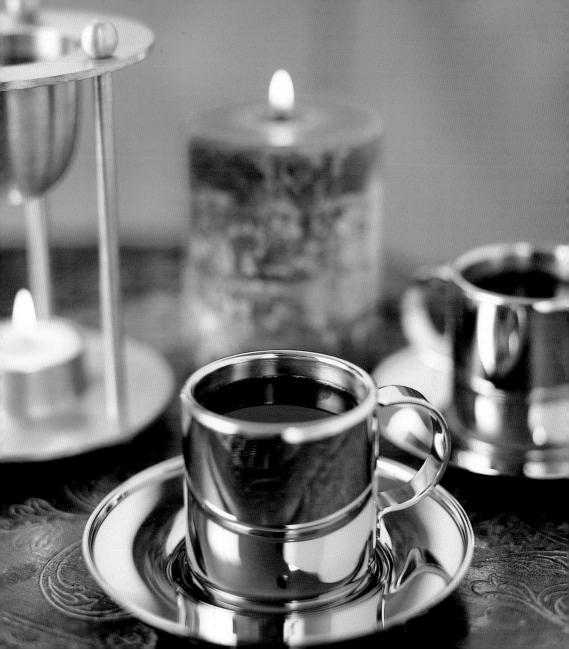

Eastern Europe

The mystery and beauty of the East is honoured here as we move towards more joy and peace. Immerse yourself in the aroma of a Bulgarian rose and feel your being soften. Create time in your life to take unknown paths and meet new people. Most of all, spend time alone, in silence, being comfortable with who you are.

Hungary

eastern festival

Held each year in Hungary to maintain friendship between Eastern European countries, the Eastern Festival helps to revive and preserve the cultures of this region. The rich and musky aroma of Angelica stimulates the same feelings of increased energy and sensuality.

2 drops Thyme
2 drops Angelica
2 drops Coriander
or
2 drops Angelica
2 drops Peppermint
2 drops Cypress

buda springs

The exotic city of Budapest in
Hungary is enlivened by the thermal
waters flowing from Buda Springs.
Wellness centres use these curative
waters in their mud baths, steam
rooms and saunas for healing
treatments. Release the same
enlivening aromas into the air and
transport your imagination to
Buda Springs.

2 drops Basil

2 drops Bergamot

2 drops Clary Sage

or

2 drops Coriander

2 drops Parsley

2 drops Thyme

hungary water

Dedicated to a 14th-century queen
of Hungary, for whom a blend of
Rosemary oil and Rosewater
(among other essential oil
ingredients) was believed to have
had incredible rejuvenating powers.
The delicate aromas of these
versions of the famous blend will
instantly lift your mood and
encourage clarity, warmth and
self-content.

2 drops Chamomile

2 drops Parsley

2 drops Rosemary

  in Rosewater

or

2 drops Bergamot

2 drops Rosemary

2 drops Juniper

  in Rosewater

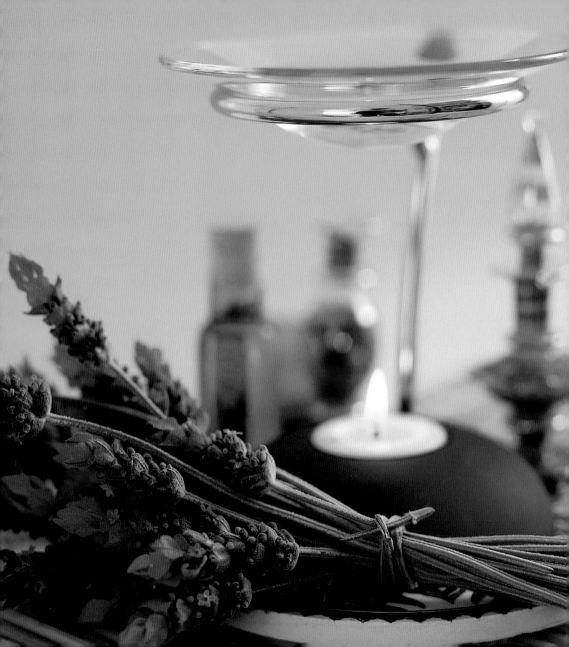

Bulgaria

valley of the roses

Bulgaria has cultivated the most superior Rose oil for the past 300 years. Distilled in the early morning from newly opened flowers, the oil symbolises innocence, love and comfort. Create a rich fragrance to strengthen the heart chakra with blends made from the essence of Bulgarian Rose blossoms.

2 drops Rose

2 drops Chamomile

2 drops Sandalwood

or

2 drops Rose

2 drops Petitgrain

2 drops Clary Sage

Czechoslovakia

city of prague

Czechoslovakia's capital of Prague attracts the vibrant European set with Art Nouveau, Baroque, Gothic and Cubist architecture, and highly creative spirit. Awaken your own creativity with these beautiful and exotic aromas reminiscent of this cosmopolitan meeting place.

2 drops Cedarwood

2 drops Bergamot

2 drops Petitgrain

or

2 drops Bergamot

2 drops Clary Sage

2 drops Lavender

Turkey

turkish bath

The traditional rejuvenation ritual, the Turkish bath—which involves dry heat, steam rooms, vigorous massage and ice-cold plunges—is taken to keep the body strong and stimulate circulation. These blends from the East are to help strengthen and stimulate your emotional constitution.

2 drops Damask Rose

2 drops Oregano

2 drops Sweet Thyme

or

2 drops Rose

2 drops Lavender

2 drops Neroli

azure coast

With the Black Sea above and the Mediterranean Sea below, between East and West, mosques and churches, lies the intriguing country of Turkey. Like its sparkling turquoise blue coast and exotically named cities—Izmir, Ephesus and Istanbul—these evocative aromas will inspire a sense of mystery.

2 drops Geranium

2 drops Lemon

2 drops Coriander

or

2 drops Cardamom

2 drops Rose

2 drops Ginger

blue mosque

Deliver the ultimate in elegant Eastern mystique at your next dinner party. Think Turkish mosque and palace with your food and floral arrangements, and fill the air with exotic music and these warming and indulgent aromas.

2 drops Sage

2 drops Cedarwood

2 drops Bergamot

or

2 drops Sandalwood

2 drops Clove

2 drops Petitgrain

Russia

russian euphoria

Distilled from the flowering tops of this plant cultivated in Russia, Clary Sage oil is the essence of optimism. Its comfortingly sweet and nutty scent will soothe in fearful moments and enhance serene dreams. It can also create a sense of complete euphoria.

2 drops Clary Sage

2 drops Vetiver

2 drops Ginger

or

2 drops Clary Sage

2 drops Black Pepper

2 drops Rose Geranium

velvet revolution

Create your own Velvet Revolution: get in touch with the quietness within and release all stress and worry. Essences chosen for their sedative properties to help reduce any uncertainty and insecure emotions. These essential oil combinations will assist the revolution—bringing calm, but also confidence.

2 drops Lavender

2 drops Bergamot

2 drops Rose

or

2 drops Coriander

2 drops Rosemary

2 drops Orange

ziva

Be inspired by Ziva, the Slavic goddess of all life. Inject some zest and passion into your day; get healthy, get moving and take a risk. Step outside your comfort zone with these blends and open yourself to new experiences and people.

2 drops Chamomile

2 drops Clary Sage

2 drops Geranium

or

2 drops Juniper

2 drops Ginger

2 drops Geranium

Romania

rain caller

In Romania, music and dance is used to bring life-giving rain in the annual spring Rain Caller festival. Use these wonderfully green and alive blends at times of new beginnings and when inspiration is needed just like rain.

2 drops Juniper

2 drops Parsley

2 drops Coriander

or

2 drops Hyssop

2 drops Rose

2 drops Parsley

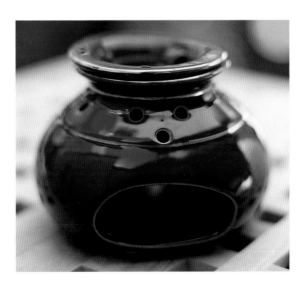

Northern Europe

In just few hours travelling through Europe, you can find a strong contrast of aromas, from the delicate scent of Lavender to the cleansing qualities of Pine. The beauty of life's journey is knowing that despite our surface differences, deep down people are the same. We are a planet of people with one heartbeat, and we have plenty of love to share.

Italy

firenze

Home to the Italian Renaissance, Florence is famous for its architecture—especially its castles and cathedrals. This city is overflowing with art. Burn these invigorating blends when you're in the mood for artistic endeavours or at the commencement of a project.

2 drops Geranium
2 drops Black Pepper
2 drops Rosemary
or
2 drops Basil
2 drops Rosemary
2 drops Lemon

juniper & tonic

Distilled from the deep blue berries of the juniper tree in Italy, Juniper essence is traditionally used to make gin—and to make a good dry martini. Known for its positive effects on the emotions, Juniper is very clearing when you're feeling negative. These blends are supportive and soothing.

2 drops Juniper

2 drops Bergamot

2 drops Myrrh

or

2 drops Juniper

2 drops Marjoram

2 drops Lime

da vinci

It is believed that legendary Italian artist Leonardo da Vinci used Neroli essential oil generously for creative inspiration. Distilled from orange blossoms, Neroli's aroma is refreshing and bitter-sweet. Known to reduce panic and fear, the Neroli in these blends will help to increase feelings of fulfilment and peacefulness.

2 drops Neroli

2 drops Clary Sage

2 drops Lavender

or

2 drops Neroli

2 drops Coriander

2 drops Ylang Ylang

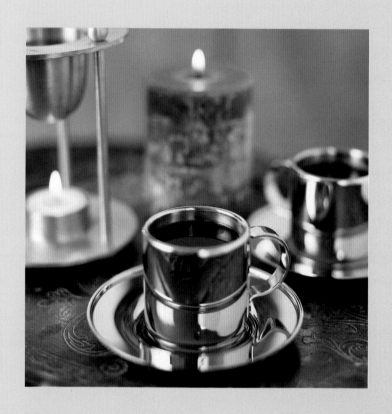

café roma

Lose yourself in the aromatic world
of authentic Italian blends:
irresistible, tempting and continental.
Capturing the essence of the Italian
café, these blends will lift the energy
of a room and add a flirtatious
touch.

2 drops Sage

2 drops Lemon

2 drops Frankincense

or

2 drops Marjoram

2 drops Thyme

2 drops Basil

bella

Blends to evoke a soft and feminine
(and decidedly Italian) quality in the
room. The feminine essence is
delicate and beautiful yet strong.
By embracing your femininity, you
can open up to powerful intuition,
love and creativity.

2 drops Mimosa

2 drops Nutmeg

2 drops Bergamot

or

2 drops Melissa

2 drops Geranium

2 drops Rose

toscana

One of Italy's most enchanted landscapes, Tuscany stretches from the mountains to the sea. Pisa and Siena beckon. Recreate the fragrances of Tuscany in your own home with these blends that will enhance good feelings in all who inhale them.

2 drops Sage

2 drops Ylang Ylang

2 drops Bergamot

or

2 drops Thyme

2 drops Vetiver

2 drops Geranium

venezia

Gondolas aren't the only attraction of this incredibly beautiful city, its maze of canals creates a sense of romantic intrigue. Manufacture your own Venetian moment with these arresting blends that will keep you alert but relaxed and ready for love.

2 drops Lavender

2 drops Lemon

2 drops Rose

in Rosewater

or

2 drops Lavender

2 drops Rosemary

2 drops Neroli

in Orangeflower Water

Spain

barcelona

The Spanish port of Barcelona has an eclectic character that sets it apart. There is a dynamism and sophistication in the Gothic and Art Nouveau architecture and the blending of different cultures. These oils will create a soft and appealing ambience that is elegant and refined.

2 drops Mandarin

2 drops Cypress

2 drops Frankincense

or

2 drops Lime

2 drops Rosemary

2 drops Sandalwood

lavender harvest

Originally from the sun-drenched Mediterranean coastline, Lavender is now cultivated and distilled in the southern regions of France and elsewhere around the world. In July, the flowers are harvested and the oil is distilled from the flowering tops. Lavender is used medicinally for its relaxing powers. It releases a very soothing, sweet and delicate scent.

2 drops Lavender

2 drops Vetiver

1 drop Sage

or

2 drops Lavender

2 drops Melissa

1 drop Juniper

France

printemps

Famous for its parfum distilleries, Grasse is also filled with the fragrances of berries and cherries from the marketplace. Essences distilled in this area include Lavender, Celery, Clary Sage, Cypress, Fennel, Jasmine and Neroli. Bring the aromas of spring in the Grasse region into your realm with these essences.

2 drops Clary Sage
2 drops Neroli
2 drops Lavender
or
2 drops Jasmine
2 drops Neroli
2 drops Lavender

paris noir

Create an atmosphere of romance and extravagance with these exquisite (and expensive) blends. When you are in the mood to indulge in a luxurious night of love and intimacy, fill your room with these essences for pleasure and imagine a magic night in Paris.

2 drops Damask Rose
2 drops Patchouli
2 drops Cypress
or
2 drops Rose Otto
2 drops Orange
2 drops Geranium

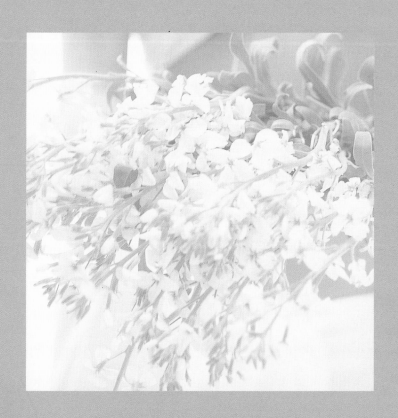

moulin rouge

Erotic and playful essences to recreate the ambience of the Moulin Rouge—the first cabaret club in Paris that attracted eccentrics, artists, musicians and aristocrats. A temple of music and hedonistic parties. These blends will boost every kind of celebration.

2 drops Sandalwood

2 drops Black Pepper

2 drops Rose

or

2 drops Ylang Ylang

2 drops Neroli

2 drops Bergamot

montparnasse

The ultimate Sunday breakfast: baguettes and coffee in a café at the Paris street markets. The atmosphere and aromas are unforgettable. Burn these calming blends on lazy Sundays when you want to lie around in bed, read the newspapers and spoil yourself.

2 drops Lavender

2 drops Sage

2 drops Bergamot

or

2 drops Coriander

2 drops Sweet Fennel

2 drops Juniper

eau de cologne

The traditional 18th-century French toilet water is still loved today for its refreshingly familiar aroma. Created with essences including Bergamot, Neroli, Lavender and Rosemary, these are recipes for clearing away unwanted odours and purifying the air.

2 drops Bergamot

2 drops Lavender

2 drops Petitgrain

in Rosewater

or

2 drops Rosemary

2 drops Neroli

2 drops Lemon

in Lavender Water

England

roman bath

The British city of Bath was founded above hot thermal springs and has a long history as a major spa town. Its incredible curative waters are enriched with an abundance of minerals. These recipes were created using the oils of plants and flowers growing in England. For inner bliss.

2 drops Peppermint

2 drops Rosemary

2 drops Orange

or

2 drops Petitgrain

2 drops Lemon

2 drops Geranium

london energy

A more upbeat blend of stimulating oils to recreate the elegant but fast-paced energy of London. There are times in our lives when we need to give ourselves an extra push to make things happen. Give everyone around a natural high with these blends.

2 drops Melissa

2 drops Grapefruit

2 drops Bergamot

or

2 drops Sweet Fennel

2 drops Lavender

2 drops Bergamot

somerset springtime

Welcome the allure of the English countryside into your room. These pleasant aromas are perfect for dinner parties. These gentle herbal blends will inspire spontaneous expressions of happiness.

2 drops Rose

2 drops Lavender

2 drops Cypress

or

2 drops Fennel

2 drops Clary Sage

2 drops Lavender

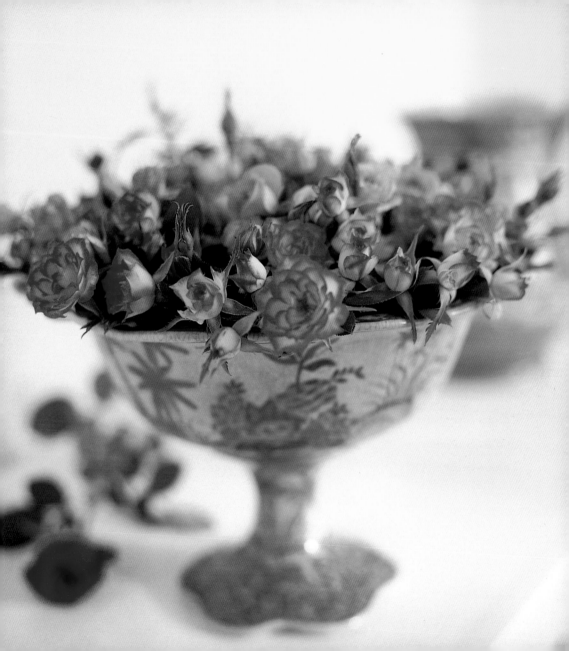

tea at the ritz

Adopt the afternoon tea tradition Londoners are fabled for. Slow down the pace and create a restful atmosphere. These potions are perfect to burn in the afternoon and early evening, and will help calm down overexcited children. Take a moment of quiet and re-energise.

2 drops Lavender
2 drops Marjoram
2 drops Chamomile

or

2 drops Lavender
2 drops Frankincense
2 drops Neroli

eau de fleurs

These divine aromas are made with floral waters—the residue of the aromatherapy distilling process. The journey of life is about finding our own balance so we can utilise our potential. Aromatherapy is just one positive way to open the mind and body to all possibilities.

2 drops Lavender
2 drops Orange
2 drops Rose
 in Rosewater

or

2 drops Lavender
2 drops Rosemary
2 drops Neroli
 in Orangeflower Water

northern lights

Seeing *aurora borealis* is an explicable wonder. Get in touch with your own wonder with deep relaxation. For extra insight, do things differently—have your lunch break at a different café, park, or go to a beach. Get a sense of your environment and enjoy the experience of watching people as they go about their day.

2 drops Pine

2 drops Rosemary

2 drops Petitgrain

or

2 drops Fir Needle

2 drops Coriander

2 drops Bergamot

belgium bathtime

A popular mineral spring, the Belgium Spa is where the whole spa phenomenon started. Burn these blends when bathing and put some spa sensations into the steamy air.

2 drops Blue Chamomile (infused)

2 drops Lavender

2 drops Neroli

or

2 drops Chamomile

2 drops Frankincense

2 drops Coriander

Holland

dutch treat

Amsterdam is the ultimate hang-out for artistic types, with fantastic galleries and cafés, and a crowd of independent-minded locals. Introduce a youthful vibe with these energising essences. Light up when you desire that free and easy feel in your day.

2 drops Patchouli

2 drops Sandalwood

2 drops Vetiver

or

2 drops Thyme

2 drops Lavender

2 drops Lemon

flower market

These enticing blends will transport your senses to the tulip and flower fields of Holland. With qualities known to enhance feelings of fulfilment and contentment, these essences are to make you feel radiant and lighter on your feet.

2 drops Mimosa

2 drops Neroli

2 drops Bergamot

or

2 drops Geranium

2 drops Juniper

2 drops Petitgrain

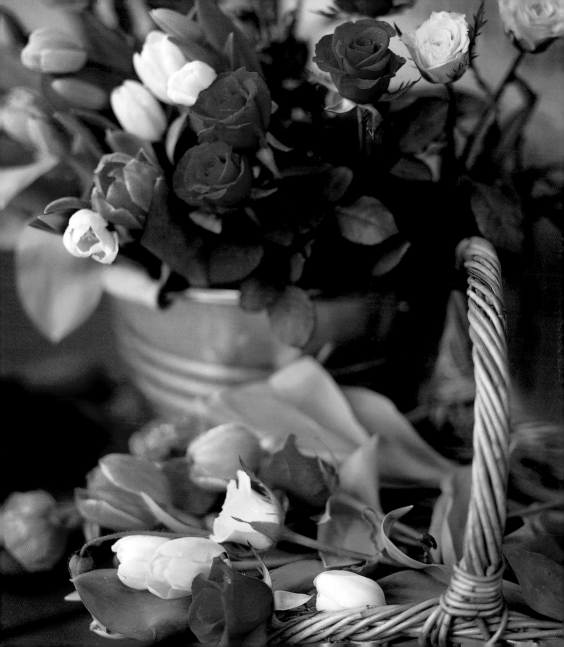

Germany

black forest

Spending a few minutes each day in nature can be transforming. Make the opportunity to get out of your head and into your body. Take a walk in an imaginary Black Forest; leave all your doubts and fears at home, stride out along the beach or through a park. These blends were created with oils to encourage vitality and endurance.

2 drops Hyssop

2 drops Geranium

2 drops Thyme

or

2 drops Fennel

2 drops Sandalwood

2 drops Lavender

berlin beat

Berlin is a European city with a unique feeling. It vibrates with interesting people and a lively nightlife. Burn these blends when you want to bring out the best in yourself and live your life to the fullest.

2 drops Cypress

2 drops Orange

2 drops Rosemary

or

2 drops Basil

2 drops Lemon

2 drops Thyme

Scandinavia

scandinavian pine

Inhale a feeling of walking through a pine forest—crispy fresh and invigorating. The essence distilled from pine needles releases a strong and fresh aroma. Historically used as an air freshener and antiseptic, Fir Needle and Pine essential oils are known to increase concentration, joy and positive emotions.

2 drops Juniper

2 drops Fir Needle

2 drops Bergamot

or

2 drops Pine

2 drops Clary Sage

2 drops Petitgrain

midnight sun

These blends are made with essences from regions around Scandinavia to celebrate the land of the midnight sun. The fresh and sweet aromas are to arouse feelings of hope and wellbeing.

2 drops Juniper

2 drops Hyssop

2 drops Peppermint

or

2 drops Hyssop

2 drops Juniper

2 drops Bergamot

South America

Spirited. Joyous.
Uninhibited. High energy.

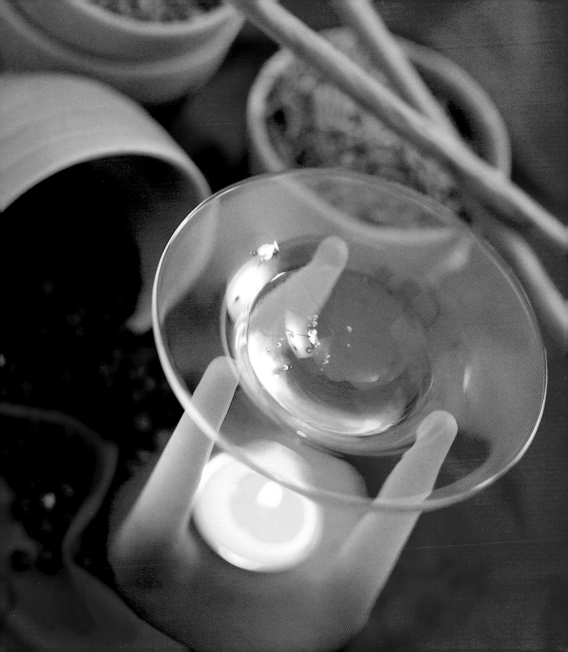

Deepen yourself by experiencing the cultures that live in the lush environments around South America. Renowned for their fiery energy, South Americans have an appealing way of expressing themselves. With these recipes, delve into the part of yourself that is wild, free and fearless.

Belize

pacha mama

The earth goddess Pacha Mama was worshipped by the ancient Incas, who had the utmost respect for Nature in all its forms—the sun, the moon, its fertility and bounty. Celebrate nature yourself with these perfect blends for spring and summer that give an aroma of fresh flowers and a new harvest.

2 drops Palma Rosa

2 drops Petitgrain

2 drops Vetiver

or

2 drops Melissa

2 drops Neroli

2 drops Chamomile

Brazil

viva brazilia

Ethnically diverse and culturally rich, Brazil is *the* place to dance the days and nights away. Burn these combos to groove with more passion and soul.

2 drops Geranium

2 drops Lime

2 drops Sandalwood

or

2 drops Rose Geranium

2 drops Ginger

2 drops Lemon Verbena

carnivale rio

It's hedonism unlimited and non-stop action at Rio's annual carnivale. The thronging crowds abandon all inhibitions, dancing and singing and partying till dawn. Create your own carnivale atmosphere with these explosive blends. They're excellent for birthdays and New Year.

2 drops Black Pepper

2 drops Lime

2 drops Cinnamon

or

2 drops Patchouli

2 drops Mandarin

2 drops Clove

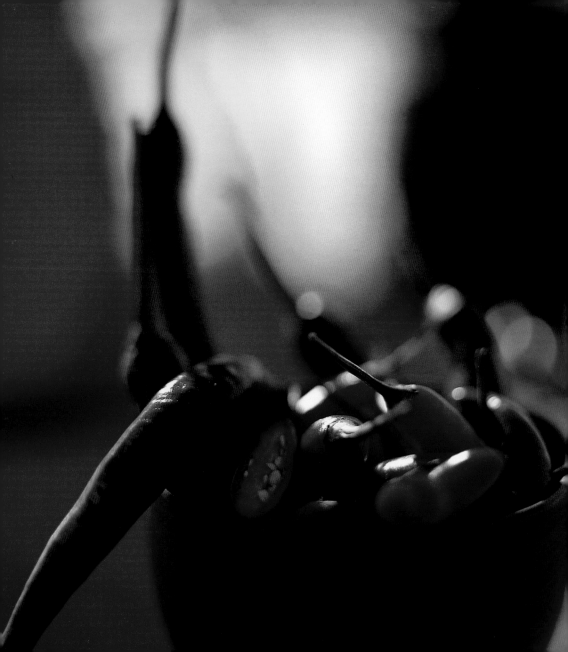

Chile

chile hot

Close to the Equator and home to some sizzling temperatures, Chile is all about having the heat turned way up. So burn these spicy blends when you want to warm up the atmosphere—before and during parties, or on a cold winter night when you desire inner contentment.

2 drops Cajuput

2 drops Ginger

2 drops Lemon

or

2 drops Rose Geranium

2 drops Sage

2 drops Fennel

Cuba

cuban rush

If your energy levels are low, inhale Cuba for an instant boost. The land of action and excitement inspired these blends, so burn them when you need extra stimulation. Ideal to increase your energy, self-confidence and motivation.

2 drops Rosemary

2 drops Basil

2 drops Coriander

or

2 drops Lemongrass

2 drops Cardamom

2 drops Petitgrain

havana hideaway

Cigars aren't the only thing Cuba's famous for. There's also its landscape of swaying palms and luscious vegetation. Evoke a faraway feeling with these sultry and smoky aromas, and take time out for some well-deserved peace and serenity.

2 drops Patchouli

2 drops Vetiver

2 drops Sandalwood

or

2 drops Cypress

2 drops Cedarwood

2 drops Cinnamon

Colombia

firewater

There's no sitting still in Colombia, home of the up-tempo salsa, danced full-speed with the aid of locally made 'Firewater'. Allow your own wild side to find expression with these energetic blends.

2 drops Basil

2 drops Lime

2 drops Ylang Ylang

or

2 drops Orange

2 drops Vetiver

2 drops Aniseed

Ecuador

spa vista

The largest spa hotel in Latin America sits on top of the Andes Mountains in Ecuador. There you can experience ancient royal healing treatments. At home, blend these invigorating essences to increase vitality and healthy emotions.

2 drops Lemongrass

2 drops Petitgrain

2 drops Clove

or

2 drops Cypress

2 drops Bergamot

2 drops Grapefruit

Jamaica

jamaican joy

Jamaicans say that their river is the place where heaven spills out into the sea. Their island home is a lush and tranquil paradise of white sands, wetlands, limestone cliffs and crystal-clear water. These blends are to create balance, even temperaments and plenty of relaxed Jamaican vibes.

2 drops Lemongrass

2 drops Petitgrain

2 drops Clove

or

2 drops Cypress

2 drops Bergamot

2 drops Grapefruit

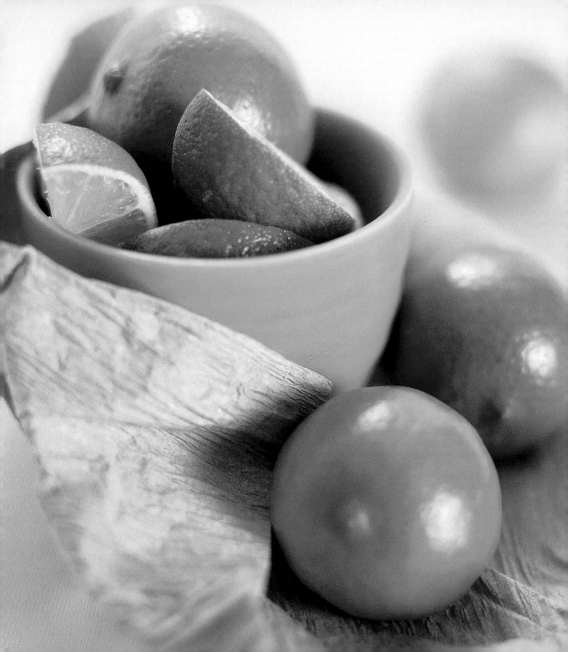

mo bay

Mo Bay, the heartland of Jamaica, is where the annual reggae Sunfest attracts a cool, bohemian crowd. Also native to Jamaica is Bay essence, with its powerful, spicy aroma. Incorporating Bay and other essential oils, these enlivening blends will add a little Jamaica to your day. These uplifting blends are made purely to brighten your mood.

2 drops Patchouli

2 drops Bay

2 drops Geranium

or

2 drops Lime

2 drops Cinnamon

2 drops Black Pepper

Mexico

lime shots

Experience the soul and colours of Mexico—vivid turquoise, pink and lime—with these fiery blends. Time for a tequila slammer or pisco sour!

2 drops Nutmeg

2 drops Lime

2 drops Orange

 in Vanilla Water

or

2 drops Sandalwood

2 drops Lime

2 drops Ginger

frida & diego

These blends were inspired by a relationship of great passion and creativity—that of the artists Frida Kahlo and Diego Rivera. Burn them when ideas are brewing and you want to bring them to the surface.

2 drops Coriander

2 drops Rosemary

2 drops Lime

or

2 drops Cypress

2 drops Basil

2 drops Lime

caribbean haven

The Caribbean is coloured by a vibrant music scene and a fusion of cultures. Liven up the atmosphere with a Caribbean beat and oils known to increase motivation. Burn these blends when you want to appreciate and enjoy the life you have been given.

2 drops Sandalwood

2 drops Patchouli

2 drops Lime

or

2 drops Juniper

2 drops Grapefruit

2 drops Ylang Ylang

Barbados

barbados

Famous for its calypso music and tiny rum stores, the island of Barbados is also home to beautiful gardens and flower forests, secluded caves and other natural treasures. This stimulating combination of essences will likewise help improve wellbeing and open your heart.

2 drops Ylang Ylang

2 drops Lime

2 drops Patchouli

or

2 drops Sandalwood

2 drops Orange

2 drops Bay

North America

Big. Bold.
Busy. Varied.

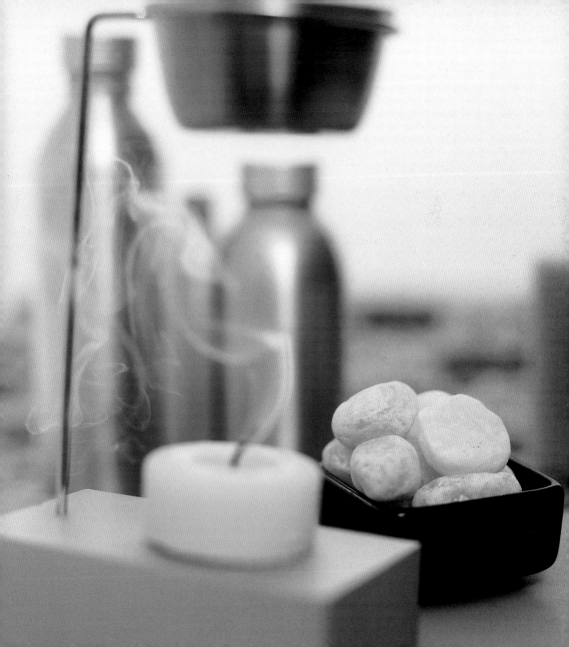

The varied aromatic blends here are to honour the true essence of this varying landscape. The mixture of cultures that epitomise America create an abundance of creative expression and an oasis of paradise for all to share.

santa fe

The desert landscape of New Mexico attracts a flow of interesting people with its intensity and provocative nature. These blends capture the sense of vast, open spaces and invite you to step outside yourself and look at life in a new light.

2 drops Melissa

2 drops Cedarwood

2 drops Juniper

or

2 drops Caraway

2 drops Grapefruit

2 drops Patchouli

new orleans

The November jazz festival in the French Quarter of New Orleans is a time of non-stop celebrations in America's Deep South. Create a similarly mellow and sensual atmosphere with these smoky aromas.

2 drops Patchouli

2 drops Geranium

2 drops Clary Sage

or

2 drops Coriander

2 drops Clove

2 drops Sandalwood

memphis blues

All the great notes come together in these melodic concoctions inspired by the musical town in Tennessee: swing, the blues, gospel and rock. Nourish yourself and those you love with some soul food. Burn the midnight oil and groove.

2 drops Vetiver

2 drops Neroli

2 drops Geranium

or

2 drops Black Pepper

2 drops Rose

2 drops Fennel

hot vapours

The sweat lodge has an important role in Native American culture. More than a physical cleansing process, the hot vapours affect your spirit, taking you to a place within where you can let go of the past and move forward. Burn these blends in times of transition: the journey inward is often the way to self-growth.

2 drops Juniper

2 drops Sage

2 drops Rosemary

or

2 drops Clary Sage

2 drops Thyme

2 drops Juniper

new york new york

The centre of the universe for movers, shakers and deal-makers, New York is a full-speed-ahead kind of place. Burn these rejuvenating essences when you need a rush of adrenaline for the day. Known to stimulate mental acuity and increase inspiration.

2 drops Lavender

2 drops Ylang Ylang

2 drops Cinnamon

or

2 drops Petitgrain

2 drops Geranium

2 drops Patchouli

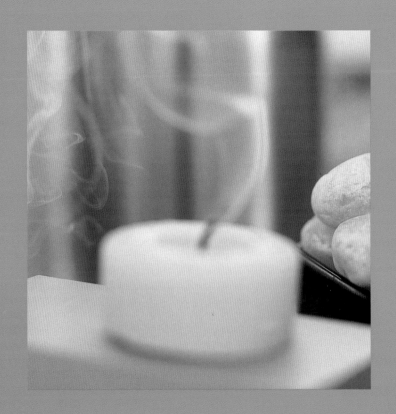

soho

Join the creative set of New York's Soho and get in touch with your artistic and imaginative side. We all have one, it's just a matter of setting aside some time to explore your dreams and bring this part out. Burn these stimulating essences when you want to draw on your visions to motivate your creativity.

2 drops Sandalwood

2 drops Grapefruit

2 drops Black Pepper

or

2 drops Geranium

2 drops Pine

2 drops Thyme

manhattan island

Manhattan has many faces: Chinatown, Soho, Central Park, Harlem. These blends are for the freethinking individual who's not afraid to express their crazy and spontaneous side—energising and spicy hot combinations to stir up some excitement. They're great to burn before meetings or when you have to perform on stage.

2 drops Cypress

2 drops Spearmint

2 drops Lemon

or

2 drops Rosemary

2 drops Coriander

2 drops Frankincense

californian sun

California is famous for its sunshine, beaches, good energy—and its oranges. The best Orange essences are from the USA and are cold-pressed from the peel. Releasing an aroma like a breath of sweet, fresh air, these blends will lift your energy when the heat is on.

2 drops Orange

2 drops Ginger

2 drops Sweet Marjoram

or

2 drops Orange

2 drops Vetiver

2 drops Clove

niagara falls

There's nothing quite as exhilirating and uplifting as a splash of cold water—and a giant waterfall makes a mighty splash. Recreate the sensation with pure Mint essential oils which are believed to help with concentration and mental clarity. A Mint blend is also an excellent shock remedy. Enlivening.

2 drops Rosemary

2 drops Spearmint

2 drops Lemon

or

2 drops Peppermint

2 drops Lavender

2 drops Cypress

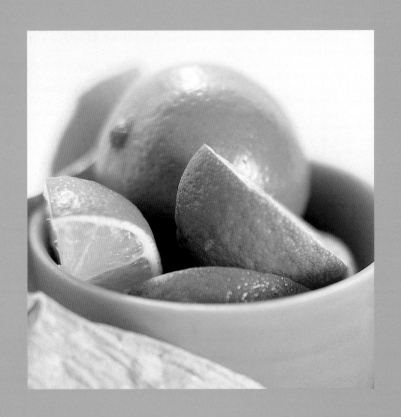

tangerine dreams

Flashback to Psychedelic America where tangerine was the colour of love and freedom. A citrus tree, the tangerine was originally cultivated in ancient China but the essence is now produced in the USA. It shares the same botanic origin as the mandarin but, because of their different growing environments, the essences are unique in fragrance. Scents of divinity, these blends are explosions of refreshing citrus to help reduce stress and lift your mood.

2 drops Mandarin

2 drops Lime

2 drops Nutmeg

or

2 drops Mandarin

2 drops Lemon

2 drops Cinnamon

bel air

Regarded as one of the best hotels in Los Angeles, the Bel Air has a swan-filled pond beside a pathway lined with a wealth of heavenly flowers. Burn these blends when you wish for material abundance in your life. The highly aromatic essences were selected to help clear decision-making and logical thought.

2 drops Jasmine

2 drops Cardamom

2 drops Cedarwood

or

2 drops Vetiver

2 drops Lime

2 drops Orange

maui spa

The Hawaiian island of Maui attracts many people interested in health and rejuvenation and the place is well known for its therapeutic treatments such as Kahuna massages, papaya enzyme baths and seaweed wraps. These blends will enhance healing, communication and emotional release. Excellent to burn while bathing.

2 drops Marjoram

2 drops Orange

2 drops Ginger

or

2 drops Cedarwood

2 drops Frankincense

2 drops Rose

san francisco

San Francisco is a vibrant city that attracts many with its diverse culture. These revitalising blends will help to start the day with a blast of good energy. Burn them, and make positive affirmations by visualising success in your projects.

2 drops Melissa

2 drops Lemongrass

2 drops Orange

or

2 drops Palma Rosa

2 drops Lime

2 drops Ginger

rocky mountain

Canada is varied in its ethnic cultures, terrain and landscape. Reflect this healthy diversity: keep yourself open and spontaneous, attempt the new, be open to change and experience variety. These blends will keep you feeling positive and in good humour.

2 drops Bergamot

2 drops Cypress

2 drops Black Pepper

or

2 drops Pine

2 drops Rosemary

2 drops Peppermint

world beat

Surrender to the beat of all cultures, people and music with blends to honour the annual Canadian World Beat festival. Sample the rhythms: Caribbean, Celtic, hip-hop, calypso, African, reggae and Latino. Spicy hot combos for everyone to enjoy.

2 drops Melissa

2 drops Black Pepper

2 drops Sandalwood

or

2 drops Mandarin

2 drops Ginger

2 drops Sandalwood

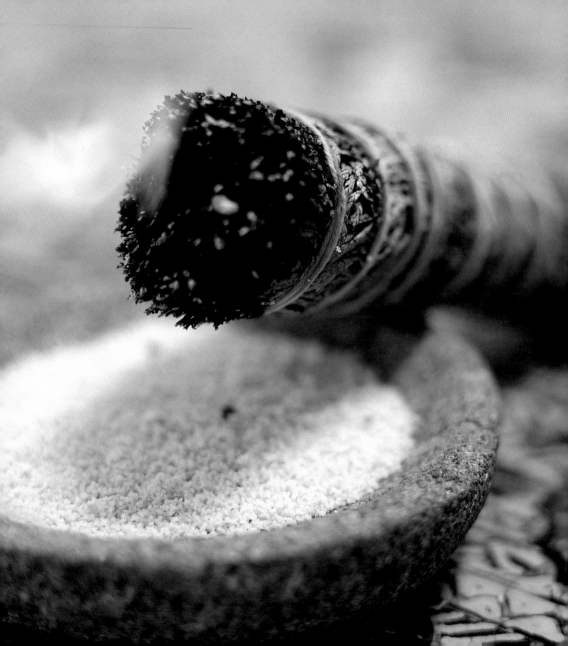

smudge stick

Many traditional cultures such as the Native Americans place great importance on cleansing ceremonies. Cleanse the air with these purifying oils when moving into a new home or office space. Other ways to start afresh are to rearrange the furniture, consult a feng shui book, and invite friends over to fill the place with a good dose of warmth and laughter.

2 drops Cinnamon

2 drops Ylang Ylang

2 drops Sage

or

2 drops Sweet Thyme

2 drops Marjoram

2 drops Rosemary

dream catcher

The energy of Native American healing rituals such as hot rock massage, drum ceremonies and desert sand paintings inspired this alchemy of potent essences. Burn them in the early evening to create calm and enhance good dreams. Take a deep breath and remember all the good things about yourself and the gifts you have to give.

2 drops Rose

2 drops Chamomile

2 drops Melissa

* in Vanilla Water*

or

2 drops Frankincense

2 drops Clary Sage

2 drops Sweet Thyme

Universal

Harmony. Union.
Awakening. Celebration.

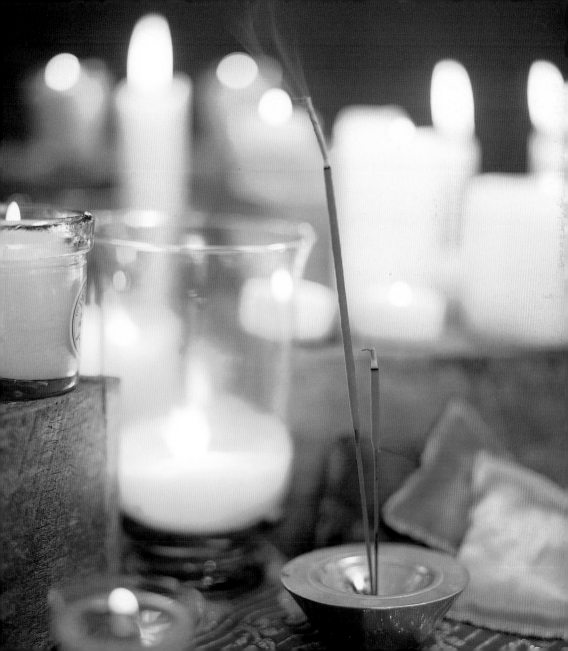

Cultures are meeting one another. People are coming together to live more harmoniously on this earth. No longer do many of us want to be divided by religion or race. An awakening is happening everywhere. We now have the self-confidence to express ourselves as we wish. These blends are to celebrate the gypsy in us all.

bohemian

The true spirit of a Bohemian is a friend who travels freely, living in the moment, loving everyone with the utmost honesty and integrity. The fire is alive in Bohemians; they bring us fresh energy. These blends celebrate personal freedom and new beginnings.

2 drops Melissa

2 drops Parsley

2 drops Hyssop

or

2 drops Lemon

2 drops Sage

2 drops Thyme

nomad

Escape the limitations of your own culture and become one with everyone who lives on this lush planet. These essences will enhance spontaneity and vitality, and assist self-empowerment. Burn them when you feel the need to relax and trust that all is happening as it should be.

2 drops Lemongrass

2 drops Orange

2 drops Cedarwood

or

2 drops Clove

2 drops Lemon

2 drops Bergamot

full moon

The full moon often brings a scattering of emotional energy and drama to your life. These blends will encourage calmness and induce better sleep. Vaporise the subtle fragrances into the night and breathe easy.

2 drops Chamomile

2 drops Geranium

2 drops Lemon-scented Eucalyptus

or

2 drops Marjoram

2 drops Juniper

2 drops Ylang Ylang

birth

Whether it is the birth of a child or a new happening in your life you are honouring, these delicate scents will lift you to a level where you can really relax and enjoy the simple things life offers. Stay strong in your truth and beauty will unfold.

2 drops Lavender

2 drops Jasmine

2 drops Sage

or

2 drops Peppermint

2 drops Lavender

2 drops Marjoram

transformation

One absolute certainty in life is that there is no certainty. Everything changes; this is one of the delights of being alive. Embracing the movement of life will keep you more joyful, and these essences were chosen to enhance wisdom and feelings of positivity and clarity.

2 drops Orange

2 drops Lime

2 drops Nutmeg

or

2 drops Ginger

2 drops Melissa

2 drops Cinnamon

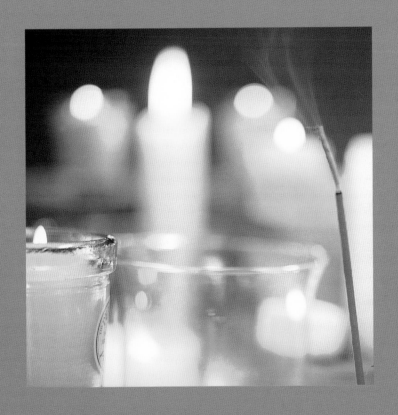

sunrise

There is nothing quite like waking up on a beautiful beach as the sun rises. Followed by a dip in the big blue ocean and what more is there left to say . . . life! Burn these warming aromas in the morning to bring happiness and love for life into the day. Enjoy!

2 drops Angelica

2 drops Sage

2 drops Bergamot

or

2 drops Rosemary

2 drops Lemon

2 drops Fennel

sunset

Take time out for yourself. A touch of silence can bring you much inner strength and joy. These aromas, known for their serene and peaceful properties, will help you let go of the day's events and take you into an evening of calm.

2 drops Cypress

2 drops Frankincense

2 drops Petitgrain

or

2 drops Juniper

2 drops Cassia

2 drops Black Pepper

emotion

All emotions are valid: joy, compassion, anger and sadness. To deny your feelings is to deny the journey of life. Use these blends when you need to take a moment to acknowledge who you are, and you will find a great love flowing from you.

2 drops Orange

2 drops Rosemary

2 drops Geranium

or

2 drops Palma Rosa

2 drops Rose Geranium

2 drops Lime

heart opener

When your heart is open, you can see the beauty in everything: nature, yourself, your friends, even people you don't normally connect with. Opening your heart can be difficult but the rewards are worthwhile. When we are in love, life is a celebration.

2 drops Geranium

2 drops Aniseed Myrtle

2 drops Cedarwood

or

2 drops Melissa

2 drops Lemon

2 drops Sandalwood

peace

Being serene is highly contagious; your easygoing presence will affect people around you in subtle yet powerful ways. Burn these essences when you feel the need to create a more tranquil environment, to bring stillness when you want to reflect awhile.

2 drops Chamomile

2 drops Frankincense

2 drops Lemon-scented Eucalyptus

or

2 drops Frankincense

2 drops Basil

2 drops Rose

meditation

It isn't always what you do in life that's significant, it's more about how you do it. Being present and caring in your attitude can give you strength and inner joy. Containing balancing properties, these blends are ideal when you want some time alone to sit, breathe and reflect.

2 drops Sandalwood

2 drops Mandarin

2 drops Nutmeg

or

2 drops Sandalwood

2 drops Vetiver

2 drops Juniper

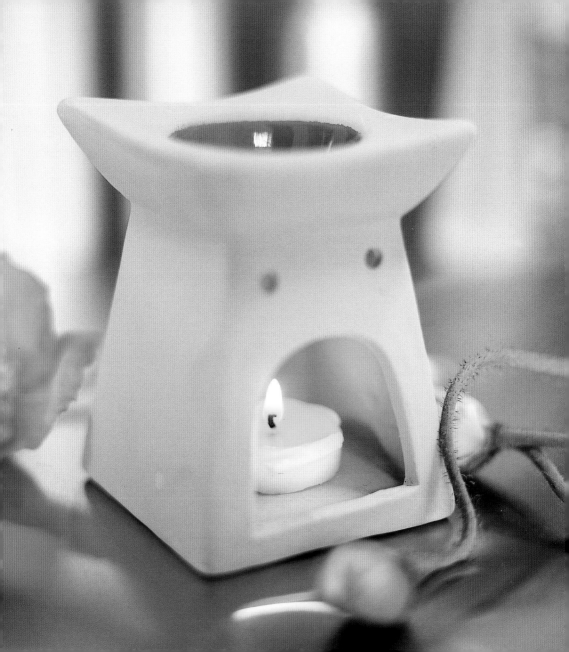

togetherness

Coming together with friends and family can be a great time of laughter and fun. The oils blended here enhance bonhomie and are excellent for increasing positivity and communication. They will create an ambience of comfort and ease.

2 drops Black Pepper

2 drops Cardomom

2 drops Jasmine

or

2 drops Patchouli

2 drops Ylang Ylang

2 drops Rose

endorphin

Release more euphoria into the atmosphere with these aromatic blends. Recognised for their mood-lifting and energy-giving properties, they are perfect when you are feeling a little low and not in full bloom.

2 drops Melissa

2 drops Peppermint

2 drops Lemon

or

2 drops Grapefruit

2 drops Ginger

2 drops Bay

rain

Rain keeps the earth lush and alive.
Burn these blends when you are
feeling stagnant, and make way for
increased clarity and purity of
thought.

2 drops Cedarwood

2 drops Clary Sage

2 drops Bergamot

or

2 drops Tea-tree

2 drops Aniseed Myrtle

2 drops Melissa

deca-dance

Dance more, laugh more, be crazy.
Don't hold back. As Tom Robbins
said: 'Humanity has advanced,
when it has advanced not because
it has been sober, responsible and
cautious, but because it has been
playful, rebellious and immature.'
Infuse these aromas at a party and
join the dance.

2 drops Grapefruit

2 drops Lemon

2 drops Geranium

or

2 drops Lemongrass

2 drops Sandalwood

2 drops Geranium

timelessness

When time seems to cease to exist, and there is nowhere special to go, you can float along with the tide with ease and grace. These essences will create a gentle calm and a feeling of playfulness. Great for lazy Sundays.

2 drops Rosemary

2 drops Pine

2 drops Thyme

or

2 drops Sweet Marjoram

2 drops Clary Sage

2 drops Melissa

benevolence

What goes around comes around. In a world that seems so off-balance sometimes, it is healthy to give and share your wealth and knowledge with others. These oil combinations are to increase vitality, warmth and openness. Reach out to those around you in any way you can.

2 drops Cinnamon

2 drops Coriander

2 drops Parsley

or

2 drops Grapefruit

2 drops Cardamom

2 drops Pine

glossary of oils

Essential oils have many properties and can be used in many different ways: in massage, baths, compresses, ointments and mouthwashes. **The blends in this book are for vaporisation only.**

Be creative and have fun with your oils, and experiment with creating your own blends. Trust your intuition!

angelica

Angelica archangelica

AVOID DURING PREGNANCY

Method of extraction	Steam distillation of the seeds
Enhances	Higher energy, inspiration, emotional strength, encouragement, support, alertness
Reduces	Fatigue, stress, respiratory problems, migraine, impatience, apathy, feelings of weakness, timidity

aniseed

Pimpinella anisum

Method of extraction	Steam distillation of the seeds
Enhances	Higher energy and rejuvenation
Reduces	Respiratory problems, mental fatigue

aniseed myrtle

Backhousia anisata

Method of extraction	Steam distillation of the leaves
Enhances	Higher energy and rejuvenation
Reduces	Respiratory problems, mental fatigue

basil

Ocimum basilicum

AVOID DURING PREGNANCY

Method of extraction	Steam distillation of the leaves and flowers
Enhances	Assertiveness, concentration, trust, happiness, purpose, balance, clarity of thought, decision-making, relaxation
Reduces	Depression, anxiety, mental fatigue, respiratory problems, scanty menstruation, loss of smell, insomnia, nervous tension, fever, nausea, hysteria, indecision

bay
Pimenta racemosa

Method of extraction	Steam distillation of the leaves
Enhances	Energy, expression, confidence, creativity, courage, the heart, sensuality
Reduces	Bronchial colds and flu, poor communication

benzoin
Styrax benzoin

USE ONLY IN SMALL AMOUNTS

Method of extraction	Resin from the bark
Enhances	Energy, calmness, confidence, protectiveness, consciousness, warmth, cleansing of air, self-empowerment, healing, openness, deep sleep, deep breathing, relaxation
Reduces	Stress, emotional exhaustion, indifference, anxiety, depression, anger, loneliness, shyness, crisis, sadness, past resentments and tensions, stagnation, respiratory problems

bergamot
Citrus bergamia

Method of extraction	Cold expression from the rind of the bergamot orange
Enhances	Positive energy, calmness, relaxation, concentration, confidence, letting go, balance, motivation, completion, joy, rejuvenation, strength, fulfilment
Reduces	Depression, anxiety, listlessness, weakened spirit, burn-out, stress, loneliness, grief, tension, bitterness, sadness

black pepper
Piper nigrum

Method of extraction	Steam distillation of the dried fruits (peppercorns)
Enhances	Clarity of thought, endurance, security, comfort, motivation, communication, direction, decision-making, aphrodisiac, confronting your fears
Reduces	Emotional blocks, anger, indecision, mental fatigue, nervousness, indifference, frustration, vagueness, stress

cajuput
Melaleuca cajuputi

Method of extraction	Steam distillation of the leaves, buds and twigs
Enhances	Higher energy, mental stimulation, centredness, wellbeing, clarity of thought
Reduces	Respiratory problems, mental fatigue, apathy, cynicism, procrastination

calendula
Calendula officinalis

Method of extraction	Infused
Enhances	Calmness, relaxation
Reduces	Inner loneliness, emotional wounds; good for children

cardamom
Elettaria cardamomum

Method of extraction	Steam distillation of the seeds
Enhances	Clarity of thought, fulfilment, concentration, confidence, motivation, sensuality, joy, caring, courage, willpower, inspiration, warming
Reduces	Stress, mental fatigue, nervous exhaustion,

thoughtlessness, uneasiness, restricted thoughts,
judgmental feelings, distrust, fear

carnation absolute

Dianthus caryophyllus

Method of extraction	Solvent extraction of the flowers
Enhances	Expression, warmth, self-esteem, imagination, trust, honesty, aphrodisiac
Reduces	Negativity, loneliness, suspicion, fear, worry, listlessness

cedarwood

Juniperus virginiana

AVOID DURING PREGNANCY

Method of extraction	Steam distillation of the wood chips and leaves
Enhances	Calmness, emotional release, positiveness, balance, sexuality, harmony, confidence, focus, security, self-empowerment, mental relaxation, emotional strength, caring, endurance
Reduces	Negativity, depression, insomnia, fear, respiratory problems, premenstrual stress, tension, vagueness, excitability, aggression, over-sensitivity, distrust, obsession, conflict

chamomile

Matricaria chamomilla (German)

Anthemis nobilis (Roman)

AVOID DURING FIRST THREE MONTHS OF PREGNANCY

Chamomile oil is very expensive, so it is more economical to buy it diluted in a carrier oil.

Method of extraction	Steam distillation of the flowers
Enhances	Healing, peace, positiveness, understanding, releasing past emotions, relaxation, stability, communication, balanced emotions, spirituality

| Reduces | Stress, depression, impatience, nerves, insomnia, hysteria, over-sensitivity, resentment |

cinnamon
Cinnamomum zeylanicum

Method of extraction	Steam distillation of the leaves
Enhances	Healing, spirituality, sensuality, awareness, security, stability, concentration, rejuvenation, warming
Reduces	Depression, mental fatigue, tension, fear, sensitivity to the hardness of life, resentment, shallowness, hatred

citronella
Cymbopogon nardus

Method of extraction	Steam distillation of the dried leaves
Enhances	Creativity, emotional strength, clarity of thought, inspiration
Reduces	Depression, lack of motivation, cluttered mind, insect repellent

clary sage
Salvia sclarea
AVOID DURING PREGNANCY

Method of extraction	Steam distillation of the leaves
Enhances	Calmness, sexuality, wellbeing, relaxation, expansion, clarity of thought, creativity, inspiration, tranquillity, balance, vitality, confidence, euphoria, communication
Reduces	Respiratory problems, irregular menstruation, nervous tension, stress, depression, migraine, over-excitement, suspicion, vagueness, fear, mental fatigue, guilt, obsessiveness, tearfulness, frigidity

clove

Eugenia caryophyllata

Method of extraction	Steam distillation of the leaves
Enhances	Mental alertness, balanced emotions, memory, endurance, security, calmness, decision-making, assertiveness, sensuality
Reduces	Mental fatigue, loss of direction, emotional weakness, feelings of failure, loss of confidence

coriander

Coriandrum sativum

Method of extraction	Steam distillation of the seeds
Enhances	Motivation, confidence, memory, communication, positive energy, creative inspiration, vitality, excitement, honesty
Reduces	Colds and flu, mental fatigue, forgetfulness, stress, nervous tension, self-doubt, frustration

cypress

Cupressus sempervirens

Method of extraction	Steam distillation of the leaves, cones and twigs
Enhances	Calmness, letting go, accepting change, strength, assertiveness, honesty, solitude, self-empowerment, inner wisdom, decisiveness, harmony
Reduces	Respiratory problems, menopausal problems, nervous tension, stress, excessive menstruation, grief, impatience, sadness, loss of direction, distrust, fear, imbalance, resentment, loneliness

eucalyptus
Eucalyptus globulus

Method of extraction	Steam distillation of the leaves
Enhances	Healing, protectiveness, concentration, vitality, balanced emotions, mental clarity, spontaneity
Reduces	Respiratory problems, fevers, headache, mental clarity, confrontations, irrational behaviour, anger, bad odours; insect repellent

fennel
Foeniculum vulgare

Method of extraction	Steam distillation of the seeds
Enhances	Happiness, perseverance, confidence, emotional release, relaxation, creativity, courage, security, rejuvenation, spirituality, assertiveness, ambition
Reduces	Loss of menstruation, nausea, menopausal problems, conflict, rigidity, fear, lack of energy and interest for life, stagnation

fir needle
Abies sibirica

Enhances	Mental stimulation, clarity, focus, emotional balance, stability
Reduces	Cold and flu symptoms, nervous tension, stressful emotions, fatigue, vagueness

frankincense
Boswellia thurifera

AVOID DURING FIRST THREE MONTHS OF PREGNANCY

Method of extraction	Steam distillation of the gum-resin
Enhances	Calmness, spirituality, balance, meditation, warming, healing, security, inner wisdom, courage, emotional release

Reduces	Respiratory problems, painful menstruation, stress, insomnia, emotional weakness, fear, exhaustion, imbalance, sorrow, dishonesty, obsession

geranium
Pelargonium graveolens

Method of extraction	Steam distillation of the leaves
Enhances	Calmness, balance, comfort, laughter, social occasions, security, self-confidence, decisiveness, logical thought, contentment, ability to change
Reduces	Menopausal problems, stress, premenstrual stress, depression, insect repellent, anxiety, lack of self-control, rigidity, mood swings, traumatic experiences both past and present, stagnation

ginger
Zingiber officinale

Method of extraction	Steam distillation of the roots
Enhances	Decisiveness, courage, confidence, strength, mental clarity, memory, sexuality, vitality, understanding, warmth, endurance
Reduces	Coughs, nausea, travel sickness, colds and flu, mental fatigue, impotence, loneliness, confusion, sadness, loss of direction, apathy

grapefruit
Citrus paradisi

Method of extraction	Steam distillation of the peel
Enhances	Balance, positive energy, confidence, joy, vitality, spontaneity, courage, security, clarity of thought, self-empowerment, inspiration, creativity, cooperation
Reduces	Depression, colds and flu, exhaustion, indecisiveness, frustration, bitterness, insecurity, sadness, irritability

hyssop

Hyssopus officinalis

Method of extraction	Steam distillation of the leaves
Enhances	Relaxation, alertness, emotional sensibility, focus
Reduces	Sluggish mind, scattered thoughts, tension, sleeplessness

jasmine

Jasminum grandiflorum

AVOID DURING PREGNANCY

Pure Jasmine oil is very expensive, so buy Jasmine oil that is diluted in a carrier oil.

Method of extraction	Solvent extraction of the flowers
Enhances	Harmony, positiveness, sexuality, self-worth, sensitivity, inspiration, clarity of thought, hope, magic, assertiveness, openness, inner wisdom, calmness, joy, warmth, romance, love
Reduces	Depression, post-natal depression, anxiety, coughs, painful menstruation, stress, premenstrual stress, apathy, lack of confidence, moodiness, bitterness, envy, emotional stagnation, frigidity

juniper

Juniperus communis

AVOID DURING PREGNANCY

Method of extraction	Steam distillation of the ripe berries
Enhances	Positiveness, healing, calmness, centredness, inner wisdom, self-confidence, fulfilment, concentration, creativity, openness, meditation, warmth
Reduces	Loss of menstruation, premenstrual stress, nervous tension, sleeplessness, anxiety, insecurity, lack of vitality

lavender

Lavandula officinalis

Method of extraction | Steam distillation of the flowers
Enhances | Calmness, balance, healing, comfort, openness, acceptance, relaxation, spirituality, resolving of conflict, strengthening, decision-making
Reduces | Depression, stress, painful menstruation, insomnia, nervous tension, migraine, premenstrual stress, emotional imbalance, fear, hysteria, frustration, shock, panic, over-sensitivity; insect repellent

lemon

Citrus limonum

Method of extraction | Cold expression from the peel
Enhances | Calmness, alertness, happiness, vitality, positiveness, laughter, motivation, decision-making, awareness, stability, ambition
Reduces | Respiratory problems, high blood pressure, forgetfulness, stress, lack of focus, apprehension, negative thoughts, bitterness, apathy, fear, mental strain, aloofness

lemon myrtle

Myrtus communis

Method of extraction | Steam distillation of the leaves
Enhances | Compassion, endurance, openness, willpower, vigour
Reduces | Intolerance, over-indulgence, lack of energy

lemon-scented eucalyptus
Eucalyptus citriodora

Method of extraction	Steam distillation of the leaves
Enhances	Healing, protectiveness, concentration, vitality, balanced emotions, mental clarity, spontaneity
Reduces	Respiratory problems, fevers, headache, mental clarity, confrontations, irrational behaviour, anger, bad odours; insect repellent

lemon verbena
Lippia citriodora

Method of extraction	Steam distillation of the flower stalks
Enhances	Concentration, motivation, joy, recovery from illness
Reduces	Apathy, stagnation, low self-esteem, unhappiness

lemongrass
Cymbopogon citratus

Method of extraction	Steam distillation of the leaves
Enhances	Concentration, vitality, awareness, clarity of thought, rejuvenation
Reduces	Depression, mental exhaustion, stress, nervousness, over-active mind

lime
Citrus aurantifolia

Method of extraction	Cold expression from the peel
Enhances	Vitality, positive energy, clarity of thought, assertiveness, decisiveness, fun, laughter, appetite for life, inspiration
Reduces	Colds and flu, depression, nervous exhaustion, stress, fatigue, self-doubt, heaviness, apathy

mandarin

Citrus nobilis

Method of extraction	Cold expression from the peel
Enhances	Inspiration, gentleness, peacefulness, empathy, emotional strength, serenity, fulfilment, motivation, encouragement
Reduces	Insomnia, nervous tension, stress, panic, past traumas, anxiety, depression, sadness, excitability, restlessness

marjoram

Origanum marjorana

AVOID DURING PREGNANCY

Method of extraction	Steam distillation of the leaves
Enhances	Restful sleep, calmness, balance, courage, determination, comfort, self-confidence, focus, warmth
Reduces	Insomnia, nervous tension, premenstrual stress, painful menstruation, colds and flu, grief, agitation, loneliness, panic, anger, resentment

melissa

Melissa officinalis

Method of extraction	Steam distillation of the leaves
Enhances	Calmness, sensitivity, happiness, harmony, positiveness, vitality, enthusiasm, alertness, security, relaxation, self-acknowledgement, confidence, hope
Reduces	Depression, feelings of emptiness, anxiety, nervous exhaustion, insomnia, respiratory problems, grief, anger, excitability

mimosa

Acacia decurrens

Method of extraction	Solvent extraction from flowers and twigs
Enhances	Joy, creativity, calm, positive outlook, restful emotions, openess, sensuality
Reduces	Dejection, closed emotions, grief, regret, aggressive thoughts, resentment, stress, menstrual tension

myrrh

Commiphora myrrha

AVOID DURING PREGNANCY

Method of extraction	Steam distillation of the gum-resin
Enhances	Spirituality, inspiration, positiveness, magic, calmness, self-assurance, letting go, rejuvenation, faith
Reduces	Respiratory problems, over-sensitivity, despair, depression, uncertainty, anger

neroli

Citrus aurantium

Method of extraction	Steam distillation of the bitter orange flowers
Enhances	Centredness, self-confidence, sensuality, positive energy, fulfilment, love, empathy, peacefulness, happiness, relaxation
Reduces	Depression, anxiety, premenstrual stress, fear, shock, panic, sorrow, past traumas, feelings of emptiness

nutmeg

Myristica fragrans

AVOID DURING PREGNANCY

Method of extraction	Steam distillation of the dried kernel (nut)

| Enhances | Enthusiasm, inspiration, playfulness, positive energy, vitality, mental stimulation, eroticism, seduction |
| Reduces | Nervousness, sexual fears, anxiety, mental exhaustion, self-doubt |

orange
Citrus aurantium

Method of extraction	Cold expression from the peel
Enhances	Sexuality, sensuality, joy, creativity, balance, self-assurance, warmth, love, communication, vitality, positive energy, balance, courage, inspiration, encouragement, consideration, pleasure
Reduces	Depression, stress, anxiety, respiratory problems, insomnia, obsession, insecurity, sadness, past traumas, emotional wounds, mental exhaustion, apathy, loss of hope

oregano
Origanum vulgare

NOT TO BE APPLIED TO SKIN

Method of extraction	Steam distilled from flowering tops
Enhances	Inner warmth and contentment, comfort, calmness, mental clarity, focus
Reduces	Hypochondriac feelings, anxiety, respiratory problems, nervous tension

palma rosa
Cymbopogon martinii

Method of extraction	Steam distillation of the dried leaves
Enhances	Clarity of thought, focus, love, vitality, balance, emotional strength
Reduces	Depression, nervous exhaustion, stress, anguish, apathy, restlessness

parsley

Petroselinum sativum

Method of extraction	Steam distillation of the seeds
Enhances	Calmness, inner strength, balanced feelings
Reduces	Nervousness, anxiety, fear, worry, menstrual tension, fever, over-sensitivity

patchouli

Pogostemon cablin

Method of extraction	Fermentation, then steam distillation of the dried leaves
Enhances	Positiveness, endurance, self-assurance, vitality, balance, consideration, gentleness, sexuality, fulfilment, purpose, laughter, wisdom, seduction, alertness, love, peacefulness
Reduces	Nervous exhaustion, stress, depression, sexual fears, insomnia, listlessness, over-sensitivity, anxiety, conflict; insect repellent

pennyroyal

Mentha pulegium

AVOID DURING PREGNANCY

Method of extraction	Steam distillation of the leaves
Enhances	Purification, positiveness, mental strength, openness, clearing
Reduces	Exhaustion, nervousness, hysteria, resentment

peppermint

Mentha piperita

AVOID DURING PREGNANCY

Method of extraction	Steam distillation of the leaves
Enhances	Concentration, vitality, self-confidence, emotional release, positiveness, sensuality, direction, clear thinking, self-empowerment
Reduces	Nausea, burn-out, shock, apathy, hysteria, colds and flu, headaches, lethargy, self-doubt, fear, vulnerabilty; insect repellent

peppermint eucalyptus

Eucalyptus dives

Method of extraction	Steam distillation of the leaves
Enhances	Healing, protectiveness, concentration, vitality, balanced emotions, mental clarity, spontaneity
Reduces	Respiratory problems, fevers, headache, mental clarity, confrontations, irrational behaviour, anger, bad odours; insect repellent

petitgrain

Citrus aurantium

Method of extraction	Steam distillation of the leaves and twigs
Enhances	Hope, calmness, harmony, communication, self-assurance, emotional strength, friendship, security, balance, inspiration, wisdom, alertness, rejuvenation, openness
Reduces	Nervous exhaustion, stress, premenstrual stress, insomnia, anxiety, vulnerability, anger, insecurity, confusion, frustration, loss of hope, sadness, stagnation

pine

Pinus sylvestris

Method of extraction	Steam distillation of pine needles and twigs
Enhances	Self-empowerment, positive energy, wisdom, trust, honesty, love, joy, focus, security, inspiration, concentration, inner strength, empathy, letting go
Reduces	Self-doubt, stress, fatigue, colds and flu, respiratory problems, frigidity, apathy, impatience, anxiety, resentment, mental fatigue, depression, guilt, sorrow, boredom, confusion

rose

Rosa centifolia

Pure Rose oil is very expensive and is best purchased diluted in a carrier oil.

Method of extraction	Solvent extraction from the rose petals
Enhances	Healing, sensuality, femininity, understanding, love, peace, passion, warmth, confidence, happiness, security, motivation, rejuvenation, openness, fulfilment, compassion
Reduces	Depression, stress, insomnia, loss of confidence, grief, apathy, insecurity, vulnerability, sexual fears, envy, feelings of emptiness, anger

rose otto

Rosa damascena

Method of extraction	Steam distillation from the damask rose
Enhances	Love, harmony, happiness, comfort, tenderness, gratitude, wisdom, spiritual awareness, confidence, sensuality, enchantment
Reduces	Despair, anxiety, sorrow, vulnerability, guilt, shyness, over-sensitivity, emotional trauma, envy, broken heart, self-doubt

rosemary

Rosmarinus officinalis

AVOID DURING PREGNANCY

Method of extraction	Steam distillation of the leaves
Enhances	Concentration, clarity of thought, warmth, emotional strength, creative inspiration, self-empowerment, centring, stability, awareness, sensuality, confidence, honesty, positive energy, decisiveness, openness, remembrance
Reduces	Mental fatigue, depression, nervous exhaustion, stress, painful menstruation, colds and flu, respiratory problems, forgetfulness, confusion, indecision, insincerity; insect repellent

sage

Salvia officinalis

AVOID DURING PREGNANCY

Method of extraction	Steam distillation of the leaves and flowers
Enhances	Healing, calmness, positiveness, balance, alertness, rejuvenation
Reduces	Depression, feelings of emptiness, anxiety, forgetfulness, fatigue, sorrow, bad odours

sandalwood

Santalum album

Method of extraction	Steam distillation of the heartwood
Enhances	Centring, openness, meditation, warmth, self-assurance, honesty, tranquillity, love, spirituality, sensuality, healing, comfort, hope, faith, inner wisdom, understanding, togetherness, stability, courage, endurance
Reduces	Depression, premenstrual stress, insomnia, stress,

sleeplessness, impotence, lack of concentration, despair, obsession, irritability, self-doubt, apprehension, scepticism, loneliness, past traumas

spearmint
Mentha spicata

Method of extraction	Steam distillation of the leaves
Enhances	Calmness, clarity, focus, compassion
Reduces	Respiratory problems, resentment, selfishness

tea-tree
Melaleuca alternifolia

Method of extraction	Steam distillation of the leaves
Enhances	Courage, confidence, mental clarity, cleansing, energising
Reduces	Colds and flu, respiratory problems, lack of confidence, scattiness

thyme
Thymus vulgaris

AVOID DURING PREGNANCY

Method of extraction	Steam distillation of the leaves and flowers
Enhances	Self-confidence, calmness, balance, focus, concentration, happiness, satisfaction, vitality, healing, determination
Reduces	Depression, fatigue, nervous exhaustion, colds and flu, fear, insomnia, anxiety; insect repellent

valerian
Valeriana officinalis

Method of extraction	Steam distillation of the root
Enhances	Calmness, happiness, emotional release, moving on,

	relaxation, deep sleep
Reduces	Stress, depression, anger, aggression, hysteria, insomnia, addiction

vanilla
Vanilla plantifolia

Enhances	Positive energy, uplifting, sensuality, romance
Reduces	Insecurity, boredom, sexual apathy

vetiver
Vetiveria zizanoides

Method of extraction	Steam distillation of the dried roots
Enhances	Wisdom, emotional release, self-confidence, centring, security, sensuality, love, comfort, emotional strength, inner wisdom, intuition, serenity
Reduces	Stress, nervous exhaustion, premenstrual stress, sleeping difficulties, over-sensitivity, vulnerability, fear, emotional burdens, scattiness, anxiety, loss of direction, stagnation, self-doubt, anger

ylang ylang
Cananga odorata

Method of extraction	Steam distillation of the flower petals
Enhances	Sensuality, exuberance, warmth, self-confidence, openness, joy, acceptance, relaxation, serenity, togetherness, tenderness
Reduces	Depression, sleeping difficulties, nervous tension, premenstrual stress, sexual inadequacy, frustration, moodiness, guilt, rigidity, thoughtlessness, broken heart

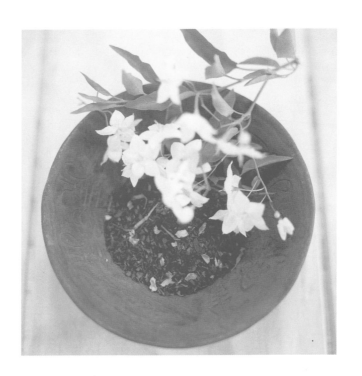

Index

Credits

The author would like to thank all the companies who lent
their products for use in the photography for this book.

cover, pages iii and 123
Oil burner from Jewels of the Earth; bowls from Made in Japan

pages vi (top) and 73
Shell bowl from Kings Queens and Soup Tureens

pages vi (middle) and 32
Stone bottle holder from Perfect Potion; oil bottles from New Directions

pages vi (bottom), 95 and 106
Oil burner from The Body Shop; candle from Kings Queens and Soup Tureens

pages vii (top), 83 and 98
Oil burner from Perfect Potion; mat from Kings Queens and Soup Tureens

pages vii (middle), 135 and 139
Oil burner from Pure Collections; stainless steel bottles from New Directions

pages vii (bottom) and 1
Oil burner from Perfect Potion

pages x (top), 149 and 153
Scent pillows from Kings Queens and Soup Tureens; candles from
Perfect Potion

pages x (middle), 63 and 77
Bottle from New Directions

pages x (bottom) and 115
Bowl and jug from Victoria Springs

pages x (bottom) and 157
Oil burner from Jewels of the Earth

page 5
Stone oil burner from Pure Collections

page 9
Oil burner from Sun Art

pages 21 and 46
Oil burner from Perfect Potion; lantern from Kings Queens and Soup Tureens

page 29
Oil burner from Pure Collections; incense burner from Kings Queens and Soup Tureens

page 35
Buddha from Jewels of the Earth; oil burner from Aveda; table runner from Kings Queens and Soup Tureens; bowl from Sun Art

page 43
Bottles from New Directions

page 55
Candle holders from Pure Collections

page 59
Rosewater bottle from Russian Empire

pages 66 and 69
Brass oil burner from Pure Collections; gold-topped bottles from Pure Magik

page 81
Bottles from New Directions

page 103
Blue oil burner from Jurlique

page 126
Purple bowl from Orson & Blake

pages 130 and 142
Turquoise bowl from Made in Japan

All herbs, spices, dried flowers, bark and roots supplied by Perfect Potion

List of suppliers of pure essential oils in Australia

ESSENTIAL THERAPEUTICS
56–60 Easy Street, Collingwood,
Victoria 3066
(03) 9419 0860

IN ESSENCE
221 Kerr Street, Fitzroy,
Victoria 3065
(03) 9486 9688
www.inessence.com.au

BLOOM PTY LTD
15-21 Cotter Street,
Richmond, Victoria 3121
(03) 9421 0200
www.bloomcosmetics.com

JURLIQUE INTERNATIONAL
PO Box 522 Oborn Road,
Mt Barker, South Australia 5251
1800 805 286
info@jurlique.com.au

ESSENTIAL SCENTS
PO Box 2096 Highett,
Victoria 2096
(03) 9553 6873
www.escents.com.au

NEW DIRECTIONS
153 Bridge Road,
Glebe, New South Wales 2037
(02) 9566 1900
www.newdirections.com.au

SPRINGFIELDS
Unit 2/2 Anella Avenue,
Castle Hill, New South Wales 2154
(02) 9894 9933
www.springfieldsaroma.com

SUNSPIRIT
6 Ti Tree Place,
Byron Bay, New South Wales 2481
1800 066 060
www.sunspirit.com.au

PERFECT POTION
Shop 5, 47 Elizabeth Street,
Brisbane, Queensland 4000
(07) 3210 0809
www.perfectpotion.com.au

THE BODY SHOP
Cnr Wellington and Jacksons Roads,
Mulgrave, Victoria 3170
1800 065 232

PURE BYRON
Shop 1, The Orient, Jonson Street,
Byron Bay, New South Wales 2481
(02) 6685 5988